OFFICE
HAZARDS

OFFICE HAZARDS

HOW YOUR JOB CAN MAKE YOU SICK

BY JOEL MAKOWER

Tilden *PRESS*

WASHINGTON, D.C.

Publisher's Note

The ideas, procedures, and suggestions contained in this book are not intended as a substitute for consulting with your physician. All matters regarding your health require medical supervision.

Printed in the United States of America

ISBN 0-9605750-0-6
Library of Congress Number 81-51116

Second Printing
February 1982

First published in 1981 by

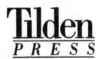

1737 DeSales Street, Northwest, Washington, D.C. 20036

_____ v

CONTENTS

The "cushy office job" has evolved into a veritable nightmare of physical and psychological ills — the stuff from which headaches and heart attacks are made.

Energy efficiency and design deficiencies have helped to make air pollution in offices a bigger health problem than air pollution outdoors. Here is a laundry list of contaminants.

When the "open" office concept hit American businesses, it hit hard. But many workers find them noisy, crowded, and uncomfortable. They may be causing more problems than they are solving.

Everyone "knows" that there's something wrong with the fluorescent lights at work, although most people aren't aware of the real problems associated with lighting in offices.

Video display terminals, a key "productivity-improving" ingredient of the automated office, are supposed to make work life easier for workers and managers, but that's far from the case.

ACKNOWLEDGEMENTS

A number of people contributed generously to this project, and they deserve recognition and thanks:

To Andrea Hricko, David LeGrande, Marsha Love, and Karen Nussbaum, all of whom supported and encouraged me during this project's early stages;

To Marian Hoffman, whose blue pencil and copy-editing skills helped to clarify and sharpen the text;

To Judith Gregory, for her endless informational resources and her comments on the first draft; and Sandra Lauffer, a fine grammarian, editor, and friend, who helped to smooth the rough edges;

To Linda Otto, for her designing and production talent; and Judith Connelly, for her sharp X-acto knife and lightning-fast paste-up ability;

To Steven Wetzler, Vernon Alt, and the staff of Mid-Atlantic Photo Composition, whose cooperation and enthusiasm made them a pleasure to work with;

To Charlene Gay, Peter Marino, Jo Molloy, Carolyn Projansky, Lorraine Rose, and Richard Spring — who variously contributed ideas, inspiration, resources, or support;

And, finally, to Shelley Liebman: for her unfailing encouragement, dedication, and assistance in every step of this project — but, most of all, for just being there.

> — *J.M.*
> *Washington, D.C.*
> *June 1981*

FOREWORD

A divorced clerical worker at the John Hancock Life Insurance Company in Boston loses custody of her child because the judge rules her full-time salary inadequate to support a family.

After nineteen years at a Cleveland bank, an office worker retires with $80 a month in pension benefits.

An administrative secretary with ten years at a Los Angeles company trains a young man to be her supervisor. He is the fourth such young man she has trained.

A school secretary with fourteen years of experience in the Minnesota school system earns less than the boy who bags her groceries at the supermarket.

Office work was once seen as a nice occupation for the woman who needed something to do before marriage; a clean alternative and a step up for the woman who would otherwise work in a factory; a pleasant environment for the woman with time on her hands and a desire for a little extra pin money.

Now the truth is coming out. Far from being the incidental job that keeps an idle woman busy, clerical work is the largest and fastest growing sector of the workforce. Yet despite its importance to the economy, such work is characterized by low pay, little promotional opportunity, and a lack of day-to-day respect — from having to get coffee for the boss, to training our own supervisors, to earning so little on full-time clerical salaries that we fall below government poverty standards.

Problems like these have spawned the working women's movement. Starting in the early 1970s, women office workers created organizations to address such issues. These organizations borrowed themes and tactics from the women's movement, the labor movement, and community organizing, and joined together into a national organization: Working Women. In Working Women we combine public action with legal action to win rights and respect. And to add to our power, we have joined with the Service Employees International Union to create a union alternative for clericals, District 925.

Over the last ten years, two factors combined to create an explosion of organizing among office workers: the growing desire for women's equality and the economic decline to the point where most families now need two incomes to meet their basic needs.

The myths of office work were shattered in the past decade. Yet office workers still counted themselves as lucky — at least the office was safe and clean, and automation would eliminate the drudgery. The mounting evidence, however, cannot be ignored. The health of office workers is threatened daily by the machines we use, the chemicals in common office products, by the design of our offices, and by the very structure of our work. A member of Working Women in Pennsylvania had her lungs virtually destroyed by exposure to a copying machine. A switchboard operator in a Cleveland insurance company developed coronary heart disease at the age of 27 after being forced to carry two workloads. An executive secretary suffered permanent hearing loss from exposure to noisy office machinery. There are many other similar examples. Joel Makower's superb book finally reveals the horrifying extent to which the office harbors health and safety hazards, and the day-to-day experiences of our members bear out his findings.

Why haven't these problems come to the surface before? What are the barriers that have kept these hazards from coming to public attention?

First, women's work in general is undervalued in this society. Since women are not considered permanent or important members of the workforce, scientists, academics,

policymakers, and employers have ignored the problems
facing women in such typically female jobs as clerical and
service work.

Second, office hazards are more subtle than most industrial hazards. The hazards work cumulatively, over
long periods of time. In some cases, scientists are just beginning to identify office hazards, and how they interact
to cause harm. More effort needs to go into such research.

In other cases, employers are well aware of hazards,
but choose to suppress the information, and that is the
third reason. For example, IBM knew for ten years that a
chemical used in one of its photocopying machines was a
suspected carcinogen. The company withdrew the product
only after independent researchers made the information
public. And studies from Europe have shown for some
time that work with video display terminals can have serious health consequences — yet employers refuse to restructure work to ease those problems.

And the future looks bad. Despite the glowing,
science-fiction-like descriptions of the office of the future,
we find that it is little more than a recreation of the factory of the past, complete with piecework, monotonous
tasks, and incredibly high rates of stress.

Alienation and health hazards of blue-collar assembly
line workers are legendary in this country. We need only
to remember the Lordstown Vega plant revolt over speed-
up in 1970; the portrayals in Studs Terkel's book, *Working*, of twenty-year veterans of steel mills who resented
every minute of their work; of the epidemic of alcoholism
on the job in order to make it through the day.

In the office, hazards from the technology itself are
coming to light almost daily, from toxics in copying machines to eyestrain and back aches from VDTs, and the
many other problems discussed in this book. These problems need to be further identified and corrected. For manufacturers to continue to market products with known
hazards is like Ford selling flammable Pintos. Such cal-
lousness and cynicism on the part of manufacturers and
management must be brought to an end.

Even more distressing are the very deep problems created by reorganizing clerical work in the modern office.

The trend is to prepare for the automated office by breaking down jobs into their smallest possible components. Clerical jobs which used to have some variety of tasks are being reorganized into eight hours a day of repeating a single task over and over. What used to be a secretary's job has become the work of data entry clerks, filers, typists, and so on. This is known as "specialization."

And it is proving to be a psychological disaster for office workers. As a result, we suffer from the second highest rate of psychological stress for 132 occupations, according to one study. Clericals working on VDTs had the highest rate of stress of all occupations, including air traffic controllers, according to another.

So, it's not only the beleaguered boss taking the worries of his $60,000-a-year job home with him who ends up with an ulcer or heart attack — it's his secretary too.

Not only is specialization bad for our health, there's no good reason for it. Recent studies show that specialization does not increase productivity. Other studies show that as work is dehumanized, productivity goes down. As jobs become more routine, as supervision is increased, as monitoring is built into machines, error rates go up. In one bank, where work was highly specialized, error rates were so high that for every check processor there was a check-processor checker. Half of the workforce was employed to check the work of the other half.

We really shouldn't be surprised by these findings. Common sense tells us that when we enjoy what we're doing, we'll do a better job. Now the scientists are verifying common sense.

No sane society — a society that placed any value on the quality of life of its working people — could knowingly create work conditions that lead to alienation and that jeopardize health. Yet that is exactly what we are doing to the nation's twenty million office workers.

These problems can be solved. The first step is to identify the problems and bring them to the light of public scrutiny. This book will be vital in doing that.

The second step is to organize. The hazards we face in offices are not individual problems; the headache that you go home with every day doesn't mean there is something wrong with *you*. On the contrary, these problems come from the machines we work with and the policies management pursues. Our work can be structured to provide variety and challenge, or it can be repetitious and monotonous. Our employers — who face many of these same hazards themselves — can provide us with machines that are safe and support research that establishes high safety standards, or they can ignore the warnings of catastrophic health impact on their workers. But such changes will come about only if we demand them.

I believe that the 1980s can be for clericals what the 1930s were for factory workers. Industrial workers were once the largest sector of the workforce, working for the most rapidly expanding sector of the economy; they were also the lowest paid, largely because they were immigrants.

We, too, are immigrants, we women who come out of the kitchens and nurseries to take up permanent places in the workforce. We're in the largest job category, and we work for enormously profitable employers. And the working conditions we face may well prove to be as perilous as those of our industrial brothers and sisters.

Just as industrial workers organized to win decent working conditions, so will office workers organize in the coming decade. And high on our agenda will be making offices safe for workers.

This book will help us to do that.

> — *Karen Nussbaum*
> *President*
> *Working Women*

THE WAY WE WORK

In scarcely more than two decades, we've transformed the office environment into an architectural and aesthetic wonderland. Cold institutional-green walls and hard tile floors have given way to rich earth tones, brightly hued panels, and plush wall-to-wall carpeting. Hard, battleship-gray furnishings have been redesigned to incorporate function with flair, even beauty. The clamor of office machinery has yielded to the soft whispers of electronic circuitry, just one indication that *efficiency* is the watchword of the day.

Who could have imagined that such handsomely engineered environments could be so incredibly hazardous to our health?

We are just beginning to pay the piper for the technological orgy of the past quarter century. There is an increasing realization that the cozy offices we've created may be as threatening to human health as are the outdoor environmental ills that have come to light during the past decade or so. The office environment threatens inhabitants with a variety of assaults from radiants, carcinogens, mutagens, allergens, noise, and other components of inadequate design — many of which are never detected by the typical worker, although they take their toll in a myriad of ways. For example:

- Office air pollution has become a major concern to health officials, as well-insulated, energy-efficient buildings combine with inadequate ventilation systems to circulate a potent mix of toxic substances like asbestos, carbon monoxide, formaldehyde, and ozone. An epidemiologist at the United Nations' World Health Organization says that "there's probably more damage to human health from indoor air pollution than from outdoor pollution."

● There's growing evidence that noise needn't be loud to be troublesome, that furniture needn't be uncomfortable to cause muscle, bone, and other physical problems, and that lighting needn't be dim to cause eyestrain. Says a researcher at the Environmental Protection Agency: "The scariest thing is that the more hidden the danger, the more serious it usually is."

● The widespread use of computers and other electronic gadgetry has introduced a whole range of problems, from tired eyes and bad backs to cataracts and cancer. Equally serious is the new brand of "stress" associated with the technology; it's linked to a large number of physical and psychological problems, not the least of which is coronary heart disease.

So much for the "cushy office job."

The office of the 1980s has become a factory, in many senses of the term. Some offices have gone into shift work, with primarily clerical workers toiling during night shifts. As in a factory, individual tasks have become "processes," each one fully analyzed and restructured to maximize efficiency. Increasingly, such processes are being automated, not unlike the assembly line. At an insurance company, for example, a claim form appears on a computer terminal screen at one workstation; the worker fills in a half-dozen elements of the form, and it automatically disappears, resurfacing at another computer terminal for additional work; meanwhile, the first worker's computer screen automatically produces another claim form — this, on and on during an eight-hour shift.

The factory-like office environment also has acquired some of the ailments of the industrial workplace: chemicals that can irritate or cause serious health problems; excessive heat and cold that can be extremely irritating, if not harmful; and disturbing amounts of physical and psychological stress caused by such things as boredom, lack of promotion opportunities, improper lighting, uncomfortable chairs, too much noise, and a host of other factors.

The factory-office link is so strong that the "office of the future" is becoming plagued with another modern-day industrial malady: expatriation of jobs. Indeed, some large-volume users of data processing and word processing ship their heavy workloads out to cheap overseas labor — in Barbados and Ireland, for example. Thanks to the miracles of telecommunications, which allows computers to talk with each other over great distances, sending and retrieving information to overseas white-collar sweatshops is as easy as dialing your telephone.

Increasingly, we are becoming a nation of white-collar factory workers. Knowledge workers — those whose work involves manipulation of symbols (like money and other numbers) or words — now make up almost half of the American work force, up from only 10 percent in 1860. Some futurists predict that by the turn of the next century, white-collar workers will constitute up to 90 percent of the work force.

Along with the growing office workplace have come growing problems for managers and executives. Productivity in the office is a central issue: overall output in offices has declined slightly in recent years, and management is fighting desperately to stop that trend. A big part of those efforts is a spate of "productivity-improving" devices and processes, from the simplest of office forms to behemoth telecommunications systems to the very walls and desks that make up the office environment. Time-study experts — now called "management consultants" — have studied the every movement of the typical secretary or clerical in an attempt to maximize the efficiency of each worker. For example, thanks to one such study, we now know that the typical secretary spends just 15 percent of the seven-hour work day typing and proofreading. Eleven percent of the time is spent on the telephone; filing and doing administrative chores consumes 21 percent of the day. The remaining 53 percent — 3 hours and 38 minutes, to be precise — is spent waiting, fetching coffee, running errands, or in other "nonproductive" activities.[1]

Of course, not everyone agrees with that analysis of secretarial efficiency. Shirley Sibert Englund, editor of _The Secretary_ magazine, reported in _Business Week_ the results of a poll taken by the National Secretary Association. That survey found that

> coffee breaks take up an average of 2.4 percent of the day; personal time (rest room visits, etc.), 2.2 percent; waiting time, 0.2 percent. Those figures, along with the 0.9 percent spent on activities having no relation to the job, add up to 5.7 percent of nonproductive time — a far cry from that harsh indictment of 53 percent, with a discrepancy of 47.3 percent. According to NSA, time consumed in productive pursuits is 94.3 percent.[2]

What has all of this quibbling to do with the hazards of office environments? Well, it seems that in the process of scrutinizing office procedures to death, there has been considerably less concern for the faces behind these numbers: the office workers. The overriding concern for the "bottom line" — not a bad concern by any means, considering the shaky nature of the economy — has obscured a great many problems. Among those problems is that many so-called productivity-improving measures may do more harm than good by causing worker discomfort or disabilities, by increasing work stress and fatigue, and by alienating workers. Ultimately, such innovations may actually *decrease* productivity, according to some experts. Part of the blame for this lies with the fact that so much of the shiny new equipment is sold primarily for its ability to improve efficiency, generally omitting the human factor. And like cars, vacations, and so many other things, office equipment is often sold to business executives as much on the basis of glamour and sex appeal as on utility.

The idea that office environments may be at all injurious to workers' well-being comes as a shock to most people, including the majority of office workers and executives. To most, "office hazards" conjures up notions of paper cuts, tripping over electrical cords, perhaps falling down the stairs. Indeed, these are hazards of office life, discussed in Chapter Seven. But there are other "office hazards" too, many of which are far more severe than a simple Band-Aid can cure.

The nature of the problem is such that the individual hazards in offices are often rather small, seemingly trivial things. Office workers rarely drop dead or lose limbs on the job. An uncomfortable chair does not seem like a major calamity; neither does stuffy air or a few ringing telephones. But put an office worker in a bad chair in a noisy, stuffy office, require that worker to perform a dead-end job for low pay on a video display terminal with a dirty screen made worse by the harsh glare from fluorescent lights, add a dash of pressure — a ruthless supervisor, for example, or economic pressures or family problems — and you've got an explosive situation, the stuff from which headaches and heart attacks are made.

The physical and psychological stresses created by office work are not particularly new; they certainly were not brought on by a handful of computers. For years, it seems, sedentary office workers have regularly encountered a veritable medical dictionary of "everyday" ailments: headaches, backaches, varicose veins, high blood pressure, deteriorating eyesight, coronary heart disease, cancers of various descriptions, and other illnesses that we have traditionally attributed to "growing old" and dismissed as unpreventable.

Amid the various disagreements and controversies that surround the issues of office environmental health, one thing is clear: Office hazards are not exclusively a secretarial or clerical problem, nor exclusively a "women's problem," although women are clearly the most frequent victims of offices' shortcomings. The same office air is breathed by men — whether executives, service and maintenance workers, or part of the growing corps of male clericals — and the inadequacies in lighting and design can make office work life more stressful than necessary for all occupants. Office hazards affect all who inhabit offices.

What's most frustrating is that virtually no one has a handle on the situation. Federal agencies traditionally concerned with the workplace — the Occupational Safety and Health Administration, the Environmental Protection Agency, the departments of Labor, and Health and Human Services — have scarcely begun to consider the problems of the office; they focus instead on the well-known horrors of industrial life. And government's role in occupational health and safety is decreasing these days; worker health and safety has been left to the devices of "the market-place." With the advent of President Ronald Reagan, the key issues surrounding occupational health and safety changed from how much the problems were hurting workers, to how much the solutions were hurting businesses. The office, it seems, is something of a regulatory no-man's land.

But the pieces are slowly beginning to emerge, as a few dozen concerned scientists, professors, researchers, and physicians have made progress in studying some of the harmful components of office life. Indeed, virtually every component of the typical office — layout, furniture, lighting, colors, windows, temperature, acoustics, graphics, even odors — is undergoing scrupulous reexamination and redesign. A veritable army of professionals in such fields as ergonomics, behavioral psychology, anthropometrics, and occupational medicine has produced a small library of literature, most of it aimed at the scientific community; *Perceptual Dimensions of Architectural Space Validated Against Behavioral Criteria* is one favorite example.

The office health and safety movement has been spurred on primarily by a growing corps of labor unions and women's groups, spearheaded by the Cleveland-based group, Working Women, a national association of office workers that has helped turn National Secretaries Week into something more than a vehicle for the American Florists Marketing Council. The coalition of feminists and labor leaders being forged during the early 1980s is creating what may well be one of the most powerful labor constituencies of the decade. With the nation's service sector growing and its industrial sector shrinking, large industrial unions — among them teamsters, auto workers, and machinists — are aiming their sights at the estimated twenty million nonunionized secretarial and clerical employees, the largest and least-organized group of workers in the country. As these workers become increasingly organized and cognizant of their rights, one certain concern will be for their health and safety.

The national office environment amounts to a massive 10.4 billion square feet — the largest physical environment after housing and manufacturing. Office space in many cities is a booming enterprise, with space renting for $30 to $70 per square foot in 1981, compared to around $10 per square foot in the same locations just six years earlier. Partly as a result of such skyrocketing costs, many businesses are moving into the growing number of cheaply (and often hastily) erected office complexes — some with no windows, bare-bones ventilation systems, and paper-thin walls. In some older cities, empty warehouses and abandoned factories are being "recaptured" for office space, with a few coats of paint and a ceilingful of fluorescent lights turning even the dingiest of places into a shiny information factory seemingly overnight. But those few improvements often obscure the fact that there may be mold growing inside the walls, soon to be causing allergies and other discomforts; that the ventilation system was designed to accommodate sacks of potatoes, not people; that rats and roaches may still be running rampant; and that there are other things needed to create productive and satisfied office workers than merely providing them with desks and chairs.

Those "other things" are what the following pages are all about. It is, admittedly, a whirlwind tour through the myriad components of the modern office environment, from the ceiling lights to the deep-rooted feelings of resentment that undermine many worker-management relationships. That resentment, it is being learned, is based not just on the nature of low-level office work — stressful, go-nowhere jobs that pay near minimum wages and provide near minimum satisfaction — but on the physical and emotional stresses such jobs create even during non-working hours; the harsh effects on mind and body that often result from performing eight hours of monotonous work at an uncomfortable and unhealthy "workstation" do not necessarily dissipate at 5 PM and on weekends.

This may not be a pleasant book to read. If you work in an office, the pages that follow may point up some things about your work environment that may be distressing, to say the least. If you manage or own such a workplace, this book may lead to a bit of rethinking — not just of your facility's physical environment, but of its entire organization, including the nature of the work itself.

The purpose of this book is not to provide the final word on office environments. That view is constantly changing, as a growing number of individuals and organizations — both in this country and abroad — try to learn more about some new aspect, however tiny, of life in the office. Rather, this book is intended to provide a starting place for understanding — a thorough statement on what we know about office environments at this point in time. It has been the lack of such a comprehensive picture that has made it difficult for workers, managers, building designers, and building owners to view office workplaces in the proper light and to take the necessary actions to solve or avoid problems.

This was written for a lay audience of workers and managers concerned about their workplaces. As such, it constantly treads a fine line between being too technical and being not sufficiently thorough. A great deal of the information is quite complex: To understand the inadequacies of fluorescent lights, for example, one needs a general background on the electromagnetic spectrum and the role of light on human health. The attempt was made to make the information as comprehensive as possible but still make it understandable to a mass audience. At the same time, it is intended that the material included here be sufficiently well documented to provide the basis for further study. In the process of striving to meet these many seemingly contradictory aims, footnotes in the text are used judiciously but, hopefully, adequately.

This is the first book written for a general audience about the hazards of office environments, but it undoubtedly will not be the last. There remains much more to be said about office work, and from many other diverse perspectives. In fact, the more we can learn, the better. If we are to become the much-talked-about nation of "knowledge workers," we'd better first apply that knowledge to creating workplaces that are as humane as they are efficient.

CHAPTER ONE

THERE'S SOMETHING IN THE AIR

Columbia Plaza, a fourteen-story office building in Washington, D.C., has made people sick almost from the start. After its completion in 1974, it was leased for twenty years to the General Services Administration, (GSA) the federal government's landlord. Within months, employees there began to realize that something was wrong.

Something is still wrong at Columbia Plaza. The building's office workers are inhabitants of a veritable torture chamber of pollutants and contaminants. For starters, exhaust fumes from the ground-level garage and loading docks circulate through the building's ventilation system, causing headaches, nausea, sleepiness, and breathing difficulties. Mold grows everywhere, giving off obnoxious odors, activating allergies, and causing respiratory problems. The heating system breaks down in winter, the air conditioning konks out in summertime. As Louise Thompkins put it, "I wouldn't be surprised if the building collapsed."

Thompkins has been a paralegal specialist for the Equal Employment Opportunity Commission for more than a decade, and with the agency moved into Columbia Plaza in 1974. The problems reached her second-floor office two years later. In the mornings, she would find herself sleepy by ten o'clock. Her supervisor sent her and others having similar problems to the agency's health unit and to other government health facilities. She was given blood tests, although she was never able to get the results, even after two years. Requests by her personal physician that she be moved to another location were ignored, until her lawyer stepped in. But even in her new location, she continued to suffer dizziness, headaches, and irregularities in her menstrual cycle.

Thompkins and the 500 or so other workers at Columbia Plaza who experienced similar difficulties are members of the American Federation of Government Employees. Union health and safety representatives complained to various government agencies, which asked GSA to solve the problems. GSA hired the Johns Hopkins University School of Public Health to study the problem. Hopkins subcontracted to an environmental testing firm, which spent a week in the building in August 1980, monitoring environmental conditions around the clock.

In December of that year, the Hopkins researchers issued a final assessment of the building, concluding primarily that "there are a high number of reports of environmental concerns and health effects." Six months later, workers there filed suit against GSA, claiming that they had received only promises and precious little action. As this book goes to press, Thompkins and others are still waiting — and wondering what effect their offices will have on their bodies over the rest of their lives.

Columbia Plaza may be extreme, but it is by no means unique. Such stories are heard almost weekly these days. Office air pollution has become a major concern to health officials — and to office workers — as well-insulated, energy-efficient buildings combine with inadequate ventilation to circulate a potent mix of toxic substances like asbestos, carbon monoxide, formaldehyde, and ozone.

Since the first concerns about "ecology" during the late 1960s, we've managed to make substantial progress in cleaning up the environment. We've established a legal network for prohibiting blatant polluting practices, established citizen groups to pressure businesses and government, and — perhaps most important — created a national consciousness that we cannot go on polluting the earth without suffering the consequences.

That movement has produced results. Outside air

quality, measured by at least three major pollutants — carbon monoxide from vehicle exhaust, sulfur dioxide from heat and electricity production, and particulate matter from soot, dust, chemicals, and metals — has steadily improved since we first became aware of "the environment." And the trend is expected to continue.

But the air inside offices is another story.

Among all of the hazards of the office, indoor air pollution may be the most severe. One reason is that, unlike other office health problems, this one is measurable; most pollutants can be detected and quantified. Another is that the effects on workers are visible, often immediate. Reports of office workers, teary-eyed and coughing, or with skin rashes resulting from irritants in the air, are appearing with a frightening frequency these days. And all indications are that the problems are going to get worse.

A few examples:

- On the sixth floor of the Simon and Schuster building in New York City's Rockefeller Center around 60 employees of NBC complained of headaches, hives, scratchy throats, and drowsiness. Investigators concluded that the newly renovated offices contained low levels of fiberglass particles that had escaped from the insulation.[1]

- In Los Angeles, 150 female workers in a new office building complained of burning eyes, coughing, breathing difficulty, nausea, lethargy, and dizziness. Employers initially shrugged off complaints, suggesting that the cause was related to pregnancy. But county health investigators found disturbing levels of formaldehyde and low levels of several other pollutants throughout the building.[2]

- A nineteen-story federal office building in Dallas had to be sealed off after employees developed a form of pneumonia that resulted from fungus in the air-conditioning system. The building was closed for two years.

- "Legionnaire's Disease," which first appeared in a Philadelphia hotel in 1976, has cropped up in office buildings throughout the country, resulting in dozens of deaths.

The list goes on and on. The problems aren't limited

either to new or old buildings. Nor are they limited to a handful of pollutants. More than a dozen chemicals capable of causing cancer, birth defects, or other serious illnesses have been identified in office environments. And there are additional substances that produce short-term irritations that can make work life unbearable.

Individually, many of these pollutants appear to be so insignificant as to be harmless. The tiny amounts of radon that can be emitted from some building materials, for example, are quite possibly harmless. But when combined with other pollutants, as well as with other physical and psychological stressors in the office, radon can prove to be a genuine menace to health. The difficulties in identifying the harmful effects of individual pollutants have been one reason why the problems of indoor air pollution have been allowed to build for so long. Another reason may be that office designers and managers haven't considered office air pollution to be a serious problem.

But a growing number of office workers do — enough, in fact, to take some pretty tough action against employers who won't listen. Unions — such as New York's Civil Service Employees Association, an affiliate of the American Federation of State, County, and Municipal Employees — have been particularly concerned with the problem. Having encountered a growing number of pollution problems in state office buildings, the union has tried to clamp down hard on workplaces that don't provide adequate air quality. "It's a serious problem," says AFSCME safety and health expert Steve Fantauzzo. "We have got to press at the bargaining table and through the grievance process to clear the air for public employees." Private-sector workers have been equally vociferous. At a 26-floor office building leased by the United Nations in New York, 900 out of 1,400 workers petitioned a government agency to look into air-quality problems. Clearly, office workers aren't taking this sitting down.

The researchers from Johns Hopkins University who investigated complaints at Washington's Columbia Plaza office building did make one fascinating revelation. While surveying Columbia Plaza's 2,000 occupants, the researchers simultaneously surveyed 500 workers in a nearby federal building from which no complaints had been received. The idea was to use the latter building as a control against which to compare Columbia Plaza. Surprisingly, the survey found that the complaints in the other building were even *higher* than in Columbia Plaza. For example: 61 percent of those at the "comparison" building complained of headaches, compared to just under 60 percent at Columbia Plaza; 54 percent complained of sinus problems, compared to 48 percent at Columbia Plaza; complaints of nasal congestion were 8 percent higher at the "comparison" building, and eye itchiness was 2 percent higher.[3] "We were really shocked," said one of the principal investigators from Hopkins. "These preliminary numbers suggest that there are many more office workers suffering in silence than we had imagined."

Ironically, many air-quality problems stem from our attempts to deal with another pressing issue: energy conservation. One major conservation effort involves sealing up buildings to decrease the amount of air that leaks out through windows, cracks, and walls. But by sealing in energy, we're also sealing in many of the pollutants that used to escape through those cracks. It's like turning a glass upside down and capturing the air. Another conservation measure is to reduce ventilation, cutting down on the need to power big, energy-draining heating and air conditioning systems. This means that the air inside a building circulates more slowly, with less fresh air coming in to sweep away the accumulating pollutants.

Still another factor is the growing number of synthetic products used inside offices: synthetic materials for carpets and drapes; plastics for machines and desks; particle board used for furniture, shelves, and space dividers; and on and on. Such materials often emit small amounts of chemicals that may be health hazards. In the past, such emissions would simply slip outside along with the other contaminants; now they're accumulating inside.

The most startling aspect of the problem is that no one really knows how polluted offices are becoming. "The work that's been done has been associated with one pollutant or another, but no one has made a comprehensive statement of the health risks we're facing indoors," says a spokesman at the U.S. Environmental Protection Agency, who preferred to remain anonymous. The field is so new, says the EPA source, and there are so many pollutants involved, that most experts agree it will take years before comprehensive information is available. But, he adds, "We can say definitely that for at least a few pollutants, there is greater risk indoors than outdoors."

That sentiment has been echoed by others. "There's probably more damage done to health by indoor air pollution than by outdoor pollution," says epidemiologist Jan Stolwijk of the World Health Organization.[4] The General Accounting Office, the investigative arm of Congress, concluded in a 1980 report, "In some cases, indoor pollution exceeds the national standards for exposure outdoors."[5] And where there's cigarette smoke, there are even more problems. According to one environmental consulting firm official, "The levels of particulate matter in office buildings where smoking is allowed is 10 to 100 times higher than the allowable limits set for outside air."[6]

Offices aren't the only places where the air is foul. Indoor air pollution is a growing concern inside homes too. But people have more control over the quality of air at home. For one thing, windows at home generally open; in most modern office buildings, they're sealed shut. For another, you can leave your home for a while without risking being fired or losing a day's pay.

A GUIDE TO OFFICE POLLUTANTS

Here's an alphabetical list of twenty major air pollutants in offices:

Ammonia. Ammonia is a colorless gas with a strong, irritating smell. It is used widely in cleaners and many other products, including some office duplicating machines, especially older ones and those used to make blueprints. Ammonia is extremely irritating, causing burning and swelling of the air passages of the nose, throat, and chest, and burning of the eyes. Not much is known about the long-term effects of ammonia.

Asbestos. This is one of the most potent killers in the office, but its effects are not generally visible. About half of all office buildings constructed between 1958 and 1970 used asbestos fibers, mostly for fireproofing and for acoustical and thermal insulation. The material was also used in many schools, restaurants, and hotels. Over the years, the asbestos fibers have begun to come loose, often circulating in building ventilation systems. In buildings that have suffered water leakage or damage or experienced high humidity levels, the asbestos deterioration is even worse.

Asbestos is a cancer-causing substance in humans. This has been known for years. What hasn't been known is how much asbestos dust causes cancer. In 1972, the Environmental Protection Agency declared asbestos a hazardous air pollutant, stating that *any* exposure to asbestos involves some health risk. In other words, no "safe" level of asbestos exposure has been determined. Environmental health officials haven't even developed accurate means for measuring asbestos concentration in the air. But whether measurable or not, it's a problem that needs to be dealt with. Crumbling acoustical tiles containing asbestos should be replaced, and air ducts or pipes containing asbestos insulation should either be removed or sprayed with a sealant to prevent further deterioration.[7] People should be evacuated from areas where asbestos repairs are being made.

Besides causing cancer of the lungs, esophagus, stomach, colon, and rectum, asbestos exposure can cause asbestosis, a chronic lung ailment; and mesothelioma, a frequently fatal form of cancer involving the thin membrane lining of the chest and abdomen.

Considering the severity of the problem, there have been precious few steps taken by those in industry and government who could help to stem the tide of asbestos-related illnesses. In its August 1980 issue, the respected *Harvard Medical School Health Letter* echoed this sentiment:[8]

> At a minimum, the federal government should be expected to take the initiative in developing a unified program to conduct research on asbestos diseases, measures to control exposures, and substitute materials. Technical advice and support should be offered to local

control programs, and a policy should be developed for the future. Asbestos diseases become a medical problem only when it is too late to cure them. Preventing these diseases is a political challenge, not a medical one.

So far, it is a challenge that remains unmet.

Benzene. This is an extremely toxic substance used in a wide variety of synthetic fibers, plastics, spot removing products, and other solvents. It is also found in tobacco smoke. In high doses, benzene acts on the central nervous system, causing drowsiness and loss of concentration. It also can affect bone marrow and blood cells, and has been found to cause chromosome damage. But even low concentrations can prove to be irritating to the liver, kidney, and gastrointestinal tract; the levels found in offices are usually extremely low. In 1980, the Occupational Safety and Health Administration set a strict new standard for benzene that was one-tenth the previous limit, although the new limit was subsequently struck down by the Supreme Court as being unreasonable. The court did not dispute the powerful nature of the chemical, however.

Cadmium. This is one of a dozen or more pollutants found in environments containing cigarette smoke (see the separate section on smoking later in this chapter). Cadmium is a highly poisonous metallic element that may cause chronic disease even in low doses. Once cadmium gets into the lungs, it's there to stay. It can damage lungs and kidneys and has been associated with emphysema and high blood pressure.

Carbon Monoxide. This is a battle that we are winning outside, but that is posing a formidable fight indoors. Carbon monoxide — known also by its chemical symbol, CO — is a colorless, odorless gas which can cause, in extreme cases, death due to asphyxiation. Its toxic effects result from being absorbed into the lungs and into the bloodstream, where it can inhibit the oxygen-carrying ability of the blood. Studies of long-term, low-dose exposures have found such symptoms as headaches, dizziness, decreased hearing, visual disturbances, personality changes, seizures, psychosis, palpitation of the heart associated with abnormal rhythms, loss of appetite, nausea, and vomiting.[9] The aged, the very young, and those with cardiac or respiratory diseases are particularly affected by carbon monoxide.

In offices, the biggest source of CO is outside air, resulting from automobile exhaust being sucked into building ventilation systems. Thus, buildings in downtown areas or along busy roadways are the ones most affected by this problem — but not exclusively. In a number of instances, underground garages and loading docks have generated high levels of carbon monoxide, which then filter up into offices.

Ethanol (also known as **ethyl alcohol**). This is contained in some duplicating fluids. It has an intoxicating effect (it is found in the fermentation process of liquor) and (like liquor) an excess of it can lead to liver damage. Other effects of inhalation include dizziness, drowsiness, and headaches, and it can dry out the skin, resulting in a scaly dermatitis.

Fiberglass. For years, this has been a primary insulation material. With the trend toward airtight buildings, however, fiberglass has emerged as a source of problems, as the tiny fibers fall from ceiling insulation or get sucked into ventilation systems without any chance of escape into the outside air.

One serious case occurred in 1980, immediately after 120 employees of the National Broadcasting Company moved into a new office on the fourth floor of the Simon and Schuster building in New York's Rockefeller Center. Within weeks, half the workers complained of hives, scratchy throats, and severe rashes. Some people had faces almost totally covered with red blotches. The culprit was fiberglass, according to the attending physician, although hired environmental consultants couldn't identify concentrations of the material in excess of standards. As it turned out, the fiberglass bags inside the ceiling were found to have broken; accurate measurements could only be taken when the ventilation system was actually blowing fiberglass-filled air out into the offices.

In addition to causing skin irritations — which are worse when the inside humidity level is low — fiberglass particles are frequently inhaled into the lungs, where they become permanently lodged.

Formaldehyde. This is another tragic case of a widely used building material that turns out to cause big problems. Formaldehyde is used in a wide variety of building materials, such as insulation, particle board, plywood, textiles, and adhesives. The $400-million-a-year formaldehyde industry produces seven million pounds of the stuff, and half of it is used in building materials. One of its principal uses in recent years has been in urea-formaldehyde foam insulation, a relatively inexpensive, easily installed, and efficient insulating material for homes and office buildings. Urea-formaldehyde foam was developed in the 1930s and became widely used in Europe in the 1960s. After limited safety studies, it was approved during the 1970s for use in the United States.

The problems stem from the fact that formaldehyde, whether in the form of insulation or as shelves or space dividers made from particle board, has a tendency to "outgas" — that is, give off fumes as it deteriorates. In an airtight office, even low levels of these fumes can cause a wide range of irritations to workers, as was clearly demonstrated in a Los Angeles office building in 1979, when 150 workers complained of burning eyes, coughing, breathing difficulties, nausea, and dizziness. Measurements showed concentrations of six to seven parts per million of formaldehyde near the walls; two parts per million is considered a legal threshold.

Those workers experienced formaldehyde's short-term effects. No one clearly understands what the long-term effects of formaldehyde are, since it hasn't been used in buildings for very long. But some serious concerns are emerging. For example, a preliminary study by the Chemical Industry Institute of Toxicology determined in 1980 that formaldehyde caused cancer in laboratory rats.[10] Such evidence helped convince the Consumer Product Safety Commission to ban further use of urea-formaldehyde foam insulation in January 1981, although as of this writing, it is doubtful that the ban will ever take effect. Massachusetts, however, is one state that has banned the use of urea-formaldehyde insulation. Meanwhile, it remains a serious threat to millions of employees working in buildings containing formaldehyde products.

Methanol. Used primarily in duplicating machine fluids, methanol can be extremely irritating to the skin, lungs, and eyes, and can affect the central nervous system. In larger doses, it can cause severe liver damage. In most office uses, however, methanol shouldn't cause problems if used in a well-ventilated area. But frequently, it isn't. For example, in the Everett School District in Washington, investigators found levels of methanol that exceeded federal standards. Nearly half the schools had no ventilation for their duplicating machines. Officials had received complaints from teacher's aides about headaches, itching eyes, and dizziness.[11] The schools removed the machines and replaced them with others.

Nitropyrenes. These are tiny yellowish crystals that are contained in small amounts in Xerox brand photocopier toners. They are not added deliberately, but may be a by-product of carbon-black production — the substance that is the "ink" of photocopies. In 1978, a Swedish researcher quietly notified Xerox that nitropyrenes had caused mutations in bacteria. Mutations in bacteria, while immediately suspect, don't necessarily cause mutations in animals or humans. After word of this finding leaked out around the world ("Tens of Thousands at Risk," trumpeted the *Western Australia Sunday Independent*), Xerox paid a visit to the Environmental Protection Agency, which issued a release advising people that they shouldn't "be alarmed about the safety of using their present copier or [about] current copying practices."[12] In March 1980, Xerox changed the formula for its toners, drastically reducing the nitropyrenes content.

There has been little study of nitropyrenes, and even that bit of research has turned up mixed conclusions about the safety of Xerox toners — and of all photocopier toners, for that matter. In the meantime, safety precautions are in order: machines should be used in well-ventilated areas, and you should avoid physical contact with the toner; if you must work with the toner, use rubber gloves and a smock and wash hands and face immediately after.

Ozone. Ozone, a colorless gas of peculiar odor, is a powerful oxidizing agent that deteriorates many materials, such as rubber, textiles, and pigments. It is an effective disinfectant, used to suppress the growth of fungus, mold, and bacteria in water supplies, industrial wastes, and foods. In high concentrations, it has a characteristic chlorine- or sulfur-like odor; in lower concentrations, it has what is often referred to as an "electric odor," also described as "pungent." Ozone also is a severe irritant to the lungs, nose, and throat. It causes inflammation of lung tissue and membranes. In addition, it causes the breakdown of red blood cells, contributes to breathing difficulties, and is suspected of producing changes in blood enzyme levels. In short, it is a deadly substance.[13]

In the office, ozone is produced when oxygen molecules come into contact with high voltages or ultraviolet light. One office machine containing both such elements is the photocopier, which can produce hazardous levels of ozone, particularly when used in a poorly ventilated room. Government standards limit ozone exposure to 0.1 parts per million for an eight-hour day, although even the National Institute for Occupational Safety and Health suggests that "...unnecessary exposure to any concentration, however small, should be avoided."[14]

In poorly ventilated areas, it is not difficult to raise ozone levels to at least twice the federal standard. A study conducted at the University of Illinois School of Public Health found that "when a photocopier was operated in a small closed room for extended periods of time, it was possible to raise indoor levels well above ambient air quality or threshold limit values." The researchers also found that "recent copying machine maintenance was found to reduce ozone production to less than detectable levels."[15] Tests conducted by NIOSH have found that grounding the photocopiers — often accomplished with a common three-pronged electrical plug — can reduce ozone emissions to tolerable levels.

Some of those NIOSH tests were conducted at the headquarters of Sperry-Univac, which manufactured three models of photocopiers (under the Remington brand) that were found to be emitting excessive levels of ozone, to the detriment of Sperry's own employees. From 1974 through 1976, Anita Reber, a secretary at Sperry-Univac's Blue Bell, Pennsylvania, facility, complained of chest pains, breathing problems, bronchitis, skin irritations, stomach pains, and various other illnesses. Her desk was located three feet from a copying machine, with the machine's exhaust facing her. Reber conducted a two-year campaign to have the situation remedied — a campaign that turned into a bitter battle culminating in a $5,000 settlement with Sperry. Meanwhile, NIOSH determined that the machines were producing hazardous amounts of ozone. NIOSH recommended that the machines "not be used in proximity to clerical and other work stations." The affected models subsequently were recalled and discontinued by Sperry.

Particulates. Any substances small enough to be inhaled into the body — dust, soot, or ash, for example — have potential for harm, since they can become deposited in the lungs. The biggest problems come from cigarette smoke, which has the tendency to gather up other particulates in the air and allow them to hang there for hours, when they might otherwise escape through ventilation exhaust systems. As stated previously, cigarette smoke can increase particulate levels by 10 to 100 times.

Polychlorinated Biphenyls (PCBs). PCBs are among the most stable of organic compounds: They do not conduct electricity, they transfer heat well, they repel water, and they are nonflammable. Primarily for these reasons, they are used widely in electrical transformers, in waterproof adhesives, in various plastics, and in carbonless carbon paper. PCBs also are virtually nondegradable and can enter the human body through a variety of means — through the skin, by inhalation, and by ingestion. By any means, they are extremely toxic, causing irritation to eyes, skin, nose, and throat, and — at high enough levels — can cause severe liver damage and are suspected of causing cancer.

There is no clear-cut evidence that PCBs are found in the office environment in normal circumstances. Carbonless carbon paper contains PCBs in tiny amounts, but it has not been shown to be a hazard. The problems with PCBs come when damage occurs to electrical transformers in office buildings. One such incident occurred in February 1981, when an explosion and fire damaged transformers in an eighteen-story state office building in

Binghamton, New York. The blast — fortunately, at 5:30 AM, when no one was in the building — spread a fine dust of PCBs throughout the building ventilation system, coating desks, files, and just about everything else. The building was closed — and will probably remain so for years, while the deadly substance is removed. The more than 700 state office workers were moved to other locations.[16] Partly as a result of a similar accident, Canada banned use of PCBs in electrical transformers.

Radon. Radon is a radioactive gas, produced by the decay of radium, which occurs naturally in a variety of substances, including rock, brick, and soil. When these substances are used in building materials, radon is emitted into the indoor environment. Radon also can enter the indoor air from radium-bearing soil underneath a building or from ground water or tap water passing through rock formations containing radium. Radon has a half-life of around 1,600 years (meaning that it loses half of its radioactivity during that period), so its presence in building materials continues for the life of the building.

Radon was never much of a concern prior to the increase in energy conservation measures; the amounts of radon that accumulated in buildings were insignificant, since most of it escaped through windows, cracks, and ventilation systems. But when fresh air is not sufficient, radon concentrations increase. The indoor radon concentration is roughly inversely proportional to the ventilation rate. In other words, cutting the ventilation level in half will approximately double the radon concentration.[17]

Unlike some of the other indoor pollutants, we have a fair amount of experience with radon, thanks to the many studies done on uranium miners in a number of countries. Those studies established a firm link between radon exposure and lung cancer. One official at the EPA estimates that as much as 10 percent of the lung cancer in the United States is caused by indoor exposure to radon. "As we seal buildings even tighter, the increased lung cancer deaths could be measured in the thousands each year," he says.

Tobacco Smoke. The effects of cigarette smoke reach smokers and nonsmokers alike, according to some recent studies. Tobacco smoke itself contains nearly 3,000 compounds — among them ammonia, benzene, formaldehyde, propane, acetylene, hydrogen sulfide, and methane — and the smoke's presence produces carbon monoxide, which interferes with the oxygen-carrying ability of blood. Moreover, cigarette smoke picks up and transports particulate matter, including dust, spores, fungi, and particles of loose fibers, such as asbestos.

More about tobacco smoke is found in the section on smoking later in this chapter.

Toluene. Like benzene, it is contained in many type-cleaning fluids and in rubber cement; like benzene, it can be dangerous if inhaled and can be an irritant when in contact with skin. Toluene is a powerful narcotic that causes sensations similar to being drunk, increasing the possibility for other accidents.

Trichloroethane. This is an organic compound that is contained in duplicating fluid. When used, its fumes are easily inhaled, which can lead to dizziness, headaches, and possible liver damage.

Trichloroethylene (TCE) (also known as **acetylene trichloride**). In high doses, this can have a depressing effect on the central nervous system and can cause liver cancer and lung dysfunction. For many years, trichloroethylene — and a very similar chemical, **tetrachloroethylene** (also known as **perchloroethylene**) — was used in well-known typewriter "white-out" formulas, in various stencil machine and typewriter cleaners, and in other office products. In 1979, a teenager in Oregon died from sniffing "Liquid Paper," and three deaths were attributed to the product in Dallas, where it is manufactured.[18] In 1979, at the urging of the Consumer Product Safety Commission, trichloroethylene was removed from product formulas, although many such products can remain in stockrooms or in use for two years or more. Moreover, CPSC has not followed up to see whether trichloroethylene is still used in other office products and has no plans to do so.

Trinitrofluorenone (TNF). This is another substance used in photocopiers that is suspected to be mutagenic — that is, capable of changing genetic material. In 1980, the IBM Corporation notified the Environmental Protection

Agency that TNF, a chemical that coats the printing drums in some IBM copier models, causes gene mutations in bacterial and mammalian cells. TNF may affect workers when it escapes from the printing drums onto copies or into the air and when the empty toner container is discarded; photocopier repair technicians are probably the ones at greatest risk. The exact nature of the problem remains undefined, while government agencies and IBM perform further tests.

Also at issue is whether IBM suppressed information about the hazards of TNF. Beginning in 1968, the company performed tests on the substance, which concluded that TNF did not produce cancer cells in mice. In a 1980 report on the subject, however, EPA reported that "this study was inadequate and the results obtained do not remove the EPA's concern for the potential carcinogenicity [cancer-causing ability] of these chemicals." In September 1980, *Computerworld* reported, "According to minutes from meetings of top IBM decision-making committees, IBM knew since before 1970 that the substance used in its photocopying process, trinitrofluorenone, is a [potential] carcinogen."[19] IBM, of course, flatly denies this. Meanwhile, the search for reliable information goes on.

Until better knowledge of photocopier hazards is found, potential problems from TNF — and other pollutants associated with photocopiers — can be minimized by using the machines in well-ventilated rooms, avoiding contact with the toners, and by having machines maintained on a regular basis.

Vinyl Chloride. This synthetic organic compound is used in a large number of plastic products. It's found in pipes, lighting fixtures, weatherstripping, furniture upholstery, wall coverings, electrical wires, laminates, and synthetic carpeting. Vinyl chloride has been a known carcinogen since the mid-1970s, and its tendency to emit vapors as it deteriorates and interacts with water and temperature changes makes it a potent indoor pollutant. Moreover, it is strongly suspected of causing gene mutations and birth defects. Other ailments linked to vinyl chloride include chronic bronchitis, ulcers, allergic dermatitis, and bone disorders.

UNDER YOUR SKIN

Air pollutants aren't the only irritants in the office. The laundry list of chemicals in the modern office also can cause a variety of skin problems — known generally as "dermatitis." In the office (or factory), such ailments are known as "occupational dermatitis." According to the National Safety Council, occupational dermatitis costs Americans more than $100 million annually in lost time and medical bills.[20]

The skin is the largest organ of the human body, encompassing about 2,900 square inches on an average person. It is also the first line of defense against a vast array of "attacks" — dirt, cuts, burns, radiation, bacteria, and harsh chemicals, for example. Not all skin reacts the same to such intrusions. Factors that come into play include sex (women are more sensitive to many irritants because their skin tends to be less oily than men's), age (younger skin tends to be more sensitive), temperature (excessive perspiration makes the skin more vulnerable to damage; dry weather makes skin sensitive too), stress (it tends to exacerbate dermatitis), and cleanliness (inadequate hygiene often causes problems).

Workplace substances can cause dermatitis in two ways. Some materials, like chemicals, are direct **irritants,** which cause damage by dissolving the skin or by extracting some of its essential components. **Sensitizers,** such as formaldehyde and organic compounds found in duplicating fluids, may cause an allergic reaction or, over long periods, can make skin so sensitive that even a tiny amount of exposure to a substance will cause a rash or other reaction.

Among the lesser-known irritants are a variety of materials handled in the course of clerical paperwork: typewriter ribbons, carbon paper, paper forms, and even ordinary typing paper, for example. Ribbons, carbon paper, and carbonless paper forms (known as NCR — "no-carbon-required" — forms) contain irritants that can cling to hands or fingers and often end up reaching the eyes. **PCBs,** discussed above, are one such example. Another is **abietic acid,** used in office paper, which has been found to cause a form of dermatitis similar to eczema. Multilith paper that contains **sodium sulfonated napthalene condensate** also has been responsible for some allergic reactions.[21]

Paper products may contain a variety of other irritating substances. Kjell Wikstrom, a Swedish dermatologist, examined one woman, a 30-year-old office worker who had no history of dermatitis, and found skin lesions over many of her fingers. Wikstrom determined that typing paper was the principal cause of the problems: "She folded typing paper and placed it both in envelopes and in plastic files of the [polyvinyl chloride] type," wrote Wikstrom in *Acta Dermato-Venereologica,* a professional journal. When she stopped doing this kind of work, the skin lesions subsided.

The suspected allergen was contained in the paper's "size" — "size" is a glue-like substance used to coat or fill in pores in typing and drawing paper. One specific size, concluded Wikstrom, contained **colophony,** a rosin, which was suspected of causing the problems. He concluded that in three of 130 cases of eczema that he examined, "the provocative cause could be traced to work with such paper."[22]

Other potential irritants contained in paper include: **oxalic acid,** used particularly in making blueprints, which can burn skin and cause nails to become brittle; **potassium hydroxide** and **sodium,** both used in the making of paper, which can cause burning, skin ulceration, and loss of fingernails.[23]

WHERE THERE'S SMOKE...

There's no need to go into the medical evidence that cigarettes cause cancer in smokers. That's well known. This is about *environments* containing cigarette smoke, and the stresses they place on everyone.

First, here's some of the most recent evidence about smoking and offices:

• A study completed by two California researchers and published in 1980 in the *New England Journal of Medicine* concluded that "chronic exposure to tobacco smoke in the work environment is deleterious to the non-smoker and significantly reduces [the lungs'] small-

airways function." The researchers found that "the passive smokers not only scored significantly lower than
their non-smoking counterparts, but also fell into the
same state of impaired [lung] performance as the nonin-
halers and the light smokers."[24]

• The more you smoke, the more coffee you want, says
a researcher at Dalhousie University in Halifax, Nova
Scotia. Cigarette smoke speeds up the elimination of
caffeine and can increase the need for coffee to maintain
caffeine levels.[25] (More on the hazards of caffeine in
Chapter Six.)

• A scientist at the University of Oklahoma Health Sciences Center has evidence that smoking cigarettes may
contribute to noise-induced hearing loss by constricting
blood vessels, which decreases blood flow to the inner
ear. Noise-induced hearing loss is the most common
reason for workers' compensation claims in the United
States.[26]

• According to Ruth Winter, author of *The Scientific
Case Against Smoking*, a typical smoker inhales only
23 percent of the smoke produced by a filtered cigarette. Nonsmokers, in other words, get about three-
fourths of the smoke — enough under some conditions
to raise blood nicotine levels of nonsmoking bystanders
to as much as 20 percent of that of smokers.[28]

Increasingly, such evidence has raised the hackles of
office workers who find that their rights to clean air are
being violated as much by fellow workers as by the building or its materials. Anti-smoking campaigns in offices
have pitted worker against fellow worker, as well as
against supervisors and subordinates. Individual cru-
saders have resorted to the courts and to administrative
agencies in their attempts to claim their rights to smoke-
less office air.

The trend toward anti-smoking activism seems to be
on the rise. According to a Louis Harris survey conducted
for the Steelcase Corporation, 35 percent of office workers
smoke in their work areas, and 51 percent of their co-
workers feel that smoking should be limited to specific
areas. But the poll also found that only 6 percent of the
companies surveyed have separate areas for smokers. And
an Administrative Management Society survey found that
fewer than 2 percent of all companies have rules against

smoking in office areas. That study found that 85 percent of all companies don't have an official policy regarding the rights of smokers and nonsmokers.[29]

Labor unions have been loath to touch this sensitive area, since they have long supported workers' rights to smoke on the job. In fact, some are still fighting no-smoking rules imposed by employers, mostly in industrial settings. But that may change, as nonsmokers become more militant.

For example, Donna M. Schimp, an employee of New Jersey Bell, suffered severe allergic reactions to cigarette smoke, including nosebleeds, vision problems, headaches, and vomiting. Her complaints to her supervisors to increase ventilation or ban smoking — and her absences from work to relieve smoke-related ailments — brought her only threats from management that she might lose her job of fifteen years. In 1975, Schimp sued her employer and conducted a fierce legal and medical campaign to win her right to a smoke-free environment. The judge ordered New Jersey Bell to limit smoking to "a nonwork area presently used as a lunchroom."

The basis of his decision was that workers have a "common law right to a safe working environment." This means that even without specific laws or regulations governing smoking, workers must be protected from any hazard. The only issue, then, was whether smoking constituted a "hazard." On this, the judge concluded, "There can be no doubt that the by-products of burning tobacco are toxic and dangerous to the health of smokers and nonsmokers generally and this plaintiff in particular."[30]

Nonsmokers have won other victories. An x-ray technician in California who was allergic to smoke quit her job after her employer failed to enforce a no-smoking rule. She was entitled to unemployment insurance benefits, ruled a state court, which said that "she has good cause for rejecting work where cigarette smoke is present because such work is not 'suitable employment' since it would be injurious to her health."[31] In another case, an Iowa state court granted unemployment benefits to a woman whose health required that she work only in a smoke-and-dust-free environment.

VENTILATION AGGRAVATION

One reason why smoking will become less popular in offices has to do with a new set of ventilation guidelines issued in early 1981 by the American Society of Heating, Refrigerating, and Air Conditioning Engineers, a trade organization. ASHRAE guidelines are considered to be highly authoritative and inevitably become the basis for state and local building codes. Among other things, the new guidelines require fewer air changes in buildings where smoking is restricted.

"ASHRAE 62," as the guidelines are known, was written to meet the dual challenges of energy efficiency and improved building ventilation. It's a difficult trade-off: To improve energy efficiency, you generally have to decrease ventilation, which leads to increased pollution and general stuffiness.

ASHRAE, by addressing such problems in a purely scientific way, omitting the human factor from its new guidelines, seems to have created the worst of both worlds — a sadly typical solution to a number of office environmental problems.

Right off the bat, ASHRAE 62 defines "acceptable air quality" as "ambient air in which there are no known contaminants at harmful concentrations and with which a substantial majority (usually 80 percent) of the people do not express dissatisfaction."

There are two major problems with this definition. For one thing, there is little consensus about what constitutes a "harmful concentration" of many known contaminants. In fact, there are no standards at all for indoor air quality for many pollutants. Concentrations of smoke, carbon monoxide, or formaldehyde that may be extremely irritating to some people may not even be noticed by others. This brings up the second problem: The "80 percent" majority of satisfied air consumers seems like a fair number — after all, you can't please everyone. But then again, some people can be severely affected by a substance such as formaldehyde — leaving them wheezing and nauseous and dizzy — while others remain unfazed. Such vague definitions leave a vast amount of leeway for employers and building managers to poorly ventilate a building and still remain within the ASHRAE guidelines.

ASHRAE 62 also suggests a curious evaluation technique to determine whether air is acceptable: "In an absence of objective means to assess the acceptability of such contaminants," reads the standard, "the judgment of acceptability must necessarily derive from subjective evaluation of impartial observers. The air can be considered acceptably free of annoying contaminants if 80 percent of a panel of at least 20 untrained observers deems the air to be not objectionable under representative conditions of use and occupancy. *An observer should enter the space in the manner of a normal visitor and should render a judgment of acceptability within 15 seconds."* [emphasis added]

It is this kind of mentality that got us into this mess in the first place. Let's assume that you, an office worker, believe that there's "something in the air" that's just not right — an abundance of cigarette smoke, perhaps, or some unidentifiable fumes that you think might be giving you a headache. And let's assume that your boss or supervisor doesn't believe that there's a problem (or won't admit it), but is willing to try out ASHRAE's "subjective evaluation." First, you'll have to find at least twenty impartial observers, which could be a challenge in itself, when you stop to think about it. Then, you bring them into the space to "render a judgment of acceptability within 15 seconds." If 80 percent of the panel approves, the air is deemed "acceptable," and you're out of luck.

Fifteen seconds? Eighty percent? Dr. James E. Wood, a professor of mechanical engineering and architecture at Iowa State University and a consultant to ASHRAE 62, explains the rationale behind this technique. "Eighty percent is a number we've used traditionally at ASHRAE for thermal comfort reasons," he says. And the fifteen-second figure came from "research done on olfactory [the sense of smell] perception and adaptation. If the judgment is made within fifteen seconds, you are still able to make a decision without adaptation." In other words, once you've been in a room for fifteen seconds, your nose begins to get used to the air, even if it's "unacceptable."

But what if the air isn't "representative" during that

quarter-minute? After all, air quality changes considerably during the day and the week. Ventilation systems click on and off on a regular basis, pollutants build up over time, and the outside air that's brought inside improves and deteriorates with such things as traffic patterns and weather conditions — all of which can affect the quality of indoor air. It is naive of ASHRAE to assume that new problems automatically can be solved by old technologies; "that's the way we've always done it" is an inappropriate rationale for professionals in the 1980s.

"We're a very quantitative society," says Dr. Alfred Hellreich, a New York City dermatologist who has examined office workers experiencing reactions to pollutants in offices where the pollutants were below maximum limits. "If you say that 'more than six' causes symptoms, everyone looks for the number more than six. And if the environment has 'less than six,' it's no problem. But if you forget the numbers and look at the patients, it's a whole different story."

To its credit, ASHRAE 62 does address the smoking problem in a very big way: It recommends that outside air intake in offices where smoking is permitted be four times higher than in offices where smoking is not permitted, a strong economic incentive to ban smoking in at least some areas of the workplace. If anything can come to the rescue of choking and teary-eyed nonsmokers, this recommendation can — if it is adopted by states and localities into building codes.

This little exercise in air-quality testing neatly demonstrates the difficulties involved in setting standards, but it also points up the frustrations of office workers, who can spend eight or nine hours a day in "acceptable" air, while still experiencing a variety of ailments, all of which can make work life unbearable and substantially reduce their satisfaction and productivity. Dr. Wood recognizes these inadequacies: "It's a very, very conservative standard. If you follow the rules, the chances are pretty good that it's going be an acceptable environment. But there's not much we can do about problems like smoking and other disagreements over comfort. Those are going to have to be resolved on a social basis."

Besides, Wood and his colleagues have their hands full dealing with some pretty important *engineering* problems. Heating, ventilation, and air-conditioning systems — known in the industry by their acronym, HVAC — are lagging sadly behind other technologies in the office.

One big problem is that HVAC systems actually can *create* pollutants, a phenomenon ably demonstrated in Philadelphia's Bellevue Stratford Hotel in 1976, where the HVAC systems produced the sometimes-fatal illness that came to be known as "Legionnaire's Disease." The disease, actually a previously unidentified form of pneumonia, didn't end with that tragic week in Philadelphia, during which 29 people died out of a total of 183 cases — nor, for that matter, did it begin in Philadelphia. "Legionnaire's Disease" has been identified in previous mysterious outbreaks, including a 1965 epidemic at a mental hospital in the District of Columbia in which there were 89 cases and twelve deaths.

Another outbreak occurred in Los Angeles in 1977, affecting nine workers at the Wadsworth Veterans Administration Hospital, killing two of them. The incident was positively connected to the facility's HVAC system: the Legionnaire's bacteria originated in the air-conditioning cooling towers in the building's roof, according to the U.S. Center for Disease Control, which investigated the incident. But it was never determined whether the cooling towers acted as reservoirs where the organisms lived and reproduced or whether they temporarily harbored organisms sucked in from the outside, then blew them out again through the building ventilation ducts. There have been similar incidents in hospitals in Memphis, Tennessee, and in Burlington, Vermont.[32]

But the phenomenon isn't limited to hospitals. At the aforementioned Columbia Plaza office building in Washington, D.C., the air-conditioning system was found to be the breeding ground for a vast mélange of molds and fungi, which were subsequently distributed through ventilation ducts into the work areas. The results included severe allergic reactions to the molds, which were found to be growing everywhere, including on walls and on paper in file cabinets.

Another such case occurred in a nineteen-story, 4,000-worker federal office building in the middle of downtown Dallas. In 1974, after receiving reports of severe pneumonia-like illnesses of office workers, the General Services Administration sealed the building off — and kept it out of commission for two years. During that time, the facility was scrubbed from top to bottom to clear out what was found to be fungus that had emanated from the air-conditioning system. The air-conditioning system itself had to be removed and replaced. A more recent occurrence was at the federal government's massive Health Resources Administration building in Hyattsville, Maryland, just outside Washington, D.C. And there are about a dozen other cases each year, according to Dr. Wallace W. Rhodes, a biologist and mechanical engineer who investigated numerous such incidents while working for the Center for Disease Control in Atlanta.

"When you reduce the outside air intake, any type of microorganisms or pollutants mount up," says Rhodes. "It's just like everybody in the house taking a bath in the same bath water without changing it. That's what happens to the air when a lot of people share it and it doesn't get changed." Moreover, says Rhodes, once you're affected by a fungal organism, you become more susceptible to reactions from other airborne substances, like gaseous pollutants.

The result, as experienced by the office workers in Dallas, Hyattsville, and numerous other cities, is known as "hypersensitivity pneumonitis," an inflammation of the lungs. Simply put, hypersensitivity pneumonitis occurs in workers after repeated inhalation of any of a wide variety of organic materials. The illness is generally suspected when respiratory and other ailments occur several hours after one spends a prolonged period in the same indoor environment. A group of doctors, reporting on the Dallas case in the *American Journal of Medicine,* suggested that "hypersensitivity pneumonitis may be a frequent cause of recurrent respiratory disease." Which is to say that if you get a lot of colds, consider the office air conditioner to be highly suspect.[33]

Another form of hypersensitivity pneumonitis has

come to be known among doctors as "humidifier lung."
Among affected workers it is known as "Monday mis-
eries," since it occurs at the beginning of the work week
after the humidifier has been shut off; actually, it is most
severe on Tuesdays following a three-day weekend. The illness, as experienced by 26 of 50 workers in a section of
one large office facility, consists of flu-like symptoms —
fever, chills, headaches, coughing, indigestion — resulting from microorganisms growing in the water of the humidifier system. When the system was turned on, the tiny
critters were spread throughout the office air, affecting
any or all who breathed it. In many cases, the symptoms
did not occur until after workers returned home from an
eight-hour work day.[34]

Humidity plays an important role in air pollution in
other ways too. Skin irritants — fiberglass, for example —
have much more of an effect when the humidity is low; the
skin is dry and more sensitive to irritants. In a closed office system with windows that can't be opened, the ventilation system spends most of the year either heating or cooling in order to maintain the desired indoor temperature.
When cooling, the system removes humidity; when heating, the system blows in dry heat. In both cases, the result
is that the inside air often has less humidity than necessary for comfort.

It isn't as if adequate ventilation systems don't exist.
Over the past few decades, mechanical engineers have
been able to design systems capable of supplying such architectural marvels as New York's World Trade Center
with sufficient heat and air conditioning. But designing
the World Trade Center's system and operating it correctly
are two different matters: The *Wall Street Journal* received
an anonymous letter from a World Trade Center worker
who complained that working in her office was "like working inside a smelly bass drum."

The root of the problem lies in the relatively one-
dimensional approach to building trades education. For
example, mechanical engineers aren't taught microbiol-
ogy, and microbiologists generally never learn mechanical
engineering. And there's precious little communication between the two disciplines — that is, until it comes time for

an interdisciplinary committee to investigate the problems surrounding a particular building *after* it has developed problems.

And then, there's just plain laziness. "Cooling towers in general do not receive as much maintenance attention as I as an equipment supplier would like to see them get," says a Maryland designer and manufacturer of air conditioning cooling towers — the kind that contributed to bacterial outbreaks in Los Angeles, Dallas, and other cities. "For one reason, they're up on a building rooftop and hard to get to and people just tend to forget about the crazy things. Besides, there hasn't been much knowledge of ventilation-spread disease, so it's of little concern to most building owners." And, of course, proper maintenance takes time — and money.

All of the above problems are solvable, given the time and the inclination. But that brings up a key issue: Inclination. In most modern buildings, supervisors, managers, and executives seem to be as much to blame for indoor air pollution problems as are mechanical engineers and building maintenance personnel: In most of the more notorious office pollution cases, organizational higher-ups were the last to acknowledge the problems — long after workers had suffered, silently or otherwise, pollution-related illnesses.

One reason for this is that supervisors and executives are less likely to be affected by air pollution problems, even if they are working in the same polluted air as clerical workers. This is because there's a fairly solid relationship between work stress — which is more likely to affect clerical workers than supervisors or executives — and the effects of pollution and other office hazards (more on this later on in this chapter). The other reason why management takes so long to remedy pollution problems holds true for virtually all other workplace hazards as well: the desire to avoid liability for worker illnesses. Once a company acknowledges that the office air quality is causing ill effects, it sets itself up for additional illness claims and possible lawsuits for negligence.

The irony, of course, is that the delays in remedying the situation often cause more problems and cost more

money for businesses. "Rather than perform routine maintenance of ventilation systems, management tends to do
things on complaint," says Dr. Dean Baker, a medical offi-
cer in the hazard evaluation and technical assistance
branch of NIOSH in New York. "It's sort of brush fire
fighting — no patterns, ineffective response. I think it's
unfair to require people to have to complain to get anything done. The average person is going to tolerate a hell
of a lot of discomfort before he complains." That puts a lot
of pressure on employees to complain, says Baker, which
can have further ill effects on worker-management relationships.

Baker is one of NIOSH's team of investigators who respond to complaints — by workers or management or
building owners —about office health and safety problems. In recent years, the number of requests for inspec-
tions and assistance with office air problems has skyrock-
eted. "We've had so many requests that it has become a
real administrative problem to try and deal with them sat-
isfactorily, scientifically, and honestly," says Dr. Richard
Keenlyside, chief of the medical section of the health hazard evaluation and technical assistance branch of NIOSH
in Cincinnati. Among Keenlyside's conclusions is that
most complaints stem from a combination of actual environmental problems and psychological stress.

One of the lesser-known aspects of office environments that Keenlyside, Baker, and others at NIOSH are
looking into is called "mass psychogenic illness." The
phrase is somewhat self-evident in its roots: *mass* (a
group of people) *psycho* (mind) *genic* (born) illnesses. Or,
simply put, a group of individuals who develop illnesses
that are at least partly psychological in origin. Recently,
some behavioral scientists have referred to the phenomenon as "mass *sociogenic* illness," the idea being that contributing causes such as sexual harassment or worker-
management strains are at least as sociological as they are
psychological in origin.

Either way, the concept is not new, nor is it limited to
office environments. It originated in the industrial workplace, where it came to be known as "assembly-line hysteria." The phrase refers to situations in which groups of

people in a work environment become sick during roughly the same period, but in which no environmental cause can be found. Instead, concluded behavioral scientists who studied the incidents, the illness was thought to be caused by stress, anxiety, and psychological conflict. The symptoms experienced by affected workers tended to be nonspecific: headaches, fatigue, dizziness, nausea, muscle fatigue, breathing difficulties — in short, the wide range of ailments commonly associated with stress.

Such stress can result from noise, poor lighting, temperature, air quality, odors, boredom, job insecurity, or other aspects of job dissatisfaction. Usually a combination of these plays a role in the illnesses. The air problems, noise, or lighting aren't bad enough to cause ill effects by themselves; they simply contribute to the overall dissatisfaction. In an inspection, office air quality might pass every temperature, ventilation, and pollution test ever devised, but in conjunction with a bad chair or a nasty supervisor, a strange odor could put a dissatisfied worker over the brink — the proverbial "straw that broke the camel's back." [35]

For example: "We recently looked at a newly refurbished office building that had a lot of problems," says Dean Baker. "During the renovation, they used a certain sort of window caulking material that had a smelly, irritating effect. Within the first few days after moving in, 10 out of 35 workers in the area had symptoms that were likely to be associated with the caulking. Eventually, over the following couple of weeks, 26 out of 35 people developed two or more symptoms that were related to the first ten cases.

"What I found was that those who had four out of five of the symptoms had developed problems within two weeks after moving in. Those who had two or more symptoms developed problems around four weeks after moving in. There was a clear division between those with specific and those with nonspecific symptoms. My interpretation was that the caulking was an initiating event that caused people to have definite symptoms. Gradually, they developed into nonspecific problems that were related to more general frustrations, such as the lack of ventilation, the inability to get rid of the caulking odors, and the fact that people knew that others were getting sick from the office air."

Mass psychogenic illness is covered more fully in Chapter Six. It is brought up here to demonstrate the lack of understanding we have of office air pollution — or most other office hazards, for that matter. The point is that the problem is not always "in the air." Nor, for that matter, is it always "in the head." It's easy to point to one or the other for matters of convenience, but things usually just aren't that simple. The tendency, of course, is to blame it all on "pollution," since it's the easiest (and most popularly understood) cause. Besides, who wants to consider that the source of their ailment is *psychological*?

BEATING THE HEAT

For all the fuss over office temperature, there's little evidence that it poses a serious physical health hazard. But that doesn't mean that it isn't a problem. The amount of psychological stress and physical discomfort resulting from inadequate temperature and/or air circulation is evident in the vast number of complaints made by workers and union representatives to management and to government agencies in recent years.

The Louis Harris poll found that "good circulation of air" and "the right temperature for you" were ranked third and fourth, respectively, in importance to office worker comfort. The survey found that air circulation is especially important to workers age 40 and older and to secretaries. Similarly, "the right temperature" is especially important to women and secretaries.

At the same time, 55 percent of office workers polled reported that the temperature in their offices just wasn't right. The complaint was highest among women (63 percent), clericals (61 percent), and those who work in "bullpen" offices with no space dividers (58 percent). Just over one-third of the office workers polled reported that their offices lacked "good circulation of air."[36] (See Chapter Two for a table containing complete results of the Harris poll.)

Why the high rate of complaints? The answer, once

again, has to do primarily with energy conservation. One simple conservation measure has been to cut back on those big, energy-draining heaters, ventilators, and air conditioners. Unfortunately, such conservation techniques, however patriotic, don't necessarily take worker comfort or productivity to heart. In many cases, the occupants of such office environments have rebelled. For example, in Toledo, Ohio, workers in a Bell Telephone office conducted a two-day walkout to protest cold office temperatures.[37] At a New York City government office building, arbitrators for AFSCME Local 1549 won compensatory time off for certain employees due to inadequate building air conditioning.[38]

Fortunately, the effects of too-cold or too-hot offices are only temporary, due to the resilience of the human body. Within a wide range of temperatures — around 45° to 95° Fahrenheit (around 7° to 35° Celsius) — there is little chance of illness or other physical hazards, other than discomfort, to the average healthy person. Among older persons or individuals with heart problems or other circulatory ailments, however, such extremes may cause ill effects. Of the two extremes, heat seems to have the most serious effects, including heat rashes, fainting, heat cramps, and heat exhaustion. Most common is simple "transient heat fatigue" — the state of discomfort and psychological strain resulting from excessive heat exposure. The effect on many workers is a decrease in performance, coordination, and alertness.

Aside from the disorders directly related to heat exposure, there is some suspicion that excessive heat might make workers susceptible to other illnesses. Researchers cite numerous instances where worker visits to dispensaries increased during hot spells. And safety managers have become familiar with the range of nonspecific health complaints they hear from workers when the temperatures in offices get high.[39]

There is some evidence that women may be more susceptible than men to excessive heat. Several studies have pointed to higher body temperatures, faster pulses, and lower sweat rates in females exposed to heat. And while the maximum endurable body temperature is the same for both sexes, actual tolerance time in severe heat is shorter for women. Women are capable of effective acclimatization to heat, but their sweat rate remains lower than that of men and general discomfort seems higher.[40] But whether these signs of greater physiological strain translate into real differences in work performance has yet to be conclusively shown.

What is the ideal temperature for office work? There are no exact numbers. According to standards set in 1980 by ASHRAE, the comfort zones are expressed as broad ranges, depending upon the time of year and the relative humidity:[41]

In Winter:
- Between approximately 67° and 73° Fahrenheit (19° and 23° Celsius) with high humidity of between 70 and 80 percent.
- Between approximately 68° and 76° Fahrenheit (20° to 25° Celsius) with low humidity of between 20 and 30 percent.

In Summer:
- Between approximately 72° and 79° Fahrenheit (22° and 26° Celsius) with high humidity of between 60 and 70 percent.
- Between approximately 74° and 81° Fahrenheit (23° and 27° Celsius) with low humidity of between 15 and 20 percent.

In other words, the higher the humidity, the lower the temperature should be.

Dr. Larry Bergland, a mechanical engineer with the John B. Pierce Foundation in New Haven, Connecticut, who worked on the above standards for ASHRAE, expressed office thermal comfort in the following terms: "The temperature range in which 80 percent of the occupants with normal clothing will be comfortable is between 72° and 78° Fahrenheit (about 22° and 26° Celsius) with 50 percent relative humidity." With heavy winter clothing, the range is 67° to 74° Fahrenheit (about 19° and 23° Celsius); with light summer clothing, the range is 75° to 81° Fahrenheit (about 24° and 27° Celsius).

As is evident from the above numbers, there are no

"ideal" temperature and humidity levels. Among other things, personal preference plays a role: some people prefer being on the cool side, others slightly warm. Other variables affecting comfort besides temperature and humidity are air movement; the amount of heat or cool radiating from ceilings, floors, and walls; clothing; the number of people in the room; and the level of human activity.

Still another variable is where you sit in the office. Temperatures near windows, for example, tend to be higher than the rest of the office in summer and lower in winter. If the window is of the "old-fashioned" type that can actually be opened, there's even more of a variation. Areas near machines or computers are sometimes warmer than the rest of the office. And the proximity to a heating or air-conditioning outlet obviously plays a role. As with so many other aspects of office life, those with the most control over their environments are generally the ones most satisfied with them.

But even with maximum flexibility, there can still be problems. "We almost always find the same common factors about offices for which we get complaints," says NIOSH's Dean Baker. "The building usually does not have as many air changes as it is supposed to have. The amount of fresh air entering the building has been decreased. And there is overcrowding. You find that, in most cases, the architects designed the floor plans and the ventilation systems for a certain number of people, but after five years, there are 30 to 40 percent more working there than were planned for. It can get awfully stuffy."

CLEARING THE AIR

Solving office air problems may not be as difficult as identifying them. As should be clear by now, the sources of pollution inside are as varied as they are outside, including everything from a building's construction material to the people themselves. The hardest part, then, is ferreting out the possible pollution sources, without jumping to any premature conclusions.

With indoor air pollution a relatively new phenomenon, the science of investigation is still in its infancy. But there are a number of basic steps to go through to determine the extent and nature of your office's problems:

Keep good records. Before you call in professionals, it's important to have as much information as possible. A brief questionnaire or informal survey taken around the office might be helpful (a sample questionnaire may be found in the Appendix of this book). Among the things you need to find out are:

- The number of people affected;
- Where in the office they are located;
- The time of day, day of week, and time of year that problems occur;
- A list of specific symptoms or illnesses;
- A rough profile of workers experiencing problems, including ages and job descriptions.

Make a list of possibilities. Create a list of all possible contributors to the problems. For example:

- The number of people in the office who smoke;
- Machines of all kinds that are used in the area;
- Fluids, cleaning solutions, or other office products that might contain chemicals, and a list of their ingredients, if known;
- Possible sources of pollution outside the building;
- Materials used in office carpets, curtains, shades, and wall coverings that might attract dust or molds or contain irritating chemicals;
- Possible sources of psychological stress, including office automation equipment, worker-management problems, fast-paced work, or constant deadlines;
- Any other factors that you feel may be important.

Document medical problems. Physicians' diagnoses are always better evidence than merely vague complaints of headaches, dizziness, fatigue, and the like. The more documented the evidence, the better the case, especially if worker complaints end up in court or in arbitration. But in instances of more general complaints, or if a doctor's consultation isn't possible, the next best thing is a detailed day-by-day log kept by everyone experiencing problems.

Go through the channels. Make sure that you've made

an attempt to notify supervisors and/or building management about the problems before you call in outsiders, since
the outside consultants or government investigators will
insist that such attempts at least be made. All parties
should be given a reasonable amount of time to find the
problems and correct them. But if the problems demand
immediate attention due to serious health problems, long
waits may be neither possible nor advisable.

Consult a government agency. NIOSH is the federal
agency that has the ability to respond to inquiries about
suspected office environmental problems, although there
may be state or local agencies that are equally capable.
NIOSH's Richard Keenlyside explains his agency's procedure: "We generally go to the workplace and do a walk-
through — which involves talking to the people who are
complaining and to the people who run the building, the
supervisors, the unions — and then walk through the
building and address the questions of concern. First we
look at the heating and ventilation system and ask questions about the amount and the make-up of the outside air
that is being brought into the building and recirculated.
Then we look for obvious sources of contamination inside
and outside the workplace that might accumulate due to
poor ventilation. Then we might take measurements of air
conditions and air velocity, using sampling pumps to
draw air through filters to analyze what's in the air; sam-
ples are taken from the breathing zone via a little tube that
is clipped onto the lapel. We leave other pumps standing
around to sample the air in the area."

The end result of all this may be quite unremarkable,
with few serious contaminants ever being discovered. But
even a clean bill of health might help everyone to breathe
more easily. Problems inevitably stem from insufficient
amounts of fresh air being brought in, says Keenlyside,
although that's no small matter if you've been suffering
stuffy air for weeks or months. The solution may be as
simple as cleaning filters or keeping the system running
more hours per day.

Devise a plan of action. If the problems turn out to be

more serious, however, you've got a formidable task ahead. Solving pollution problems can be an expensive and time-consuming job; needless to say, few building owners are particularly grateful about going through the process.

If the problems are typical, it may not be possible to solve them all at once. Some solutions may require major repairs or renovations. In consultation with experts from NIOSH or another government agency, and possibly a mechanical engineer, you should devise a list of recommended solutions along with a reasonable set of priorities and a timetable for implementing them. Such a list will serve as a basis for negotiations with an employer or landlord, and might provide weight to your case should your complaints ever end up in court.

CHAPTER TWO

DESIGN NEGLECT

How well was your office designed?

The question isn't often considered consciously by office workers, although if asked, most could recite a litany of discomforts and aggravations about the design, efficiency, and comfort of their offices. Unfortunately, most office workers are never asked.

In 1980, the Louis Harris organization did ask, in an extensive poll it conducted for Steelcase Inc., a major manufacturer of office products and furniture. The pollsters presented workers and executives with a list of twelve factors affecting comfort and productivity, asking them to rank each according to importance. First and foremost was "good lighting," a subject discussed in the following chapter. The rest of the rankings are contained in the table on the next page.

A few other Harris poll findings are worth noting. Executives agreed with office workers on most aspects of design and comfort, although they ranked air circulation and temperature higher on the list than did their employees. Secretaries were much more concerned about chairs, air quality, and temperature than were executives, managers, supervisors, and professional workers. Factors most frequently mentioned as lacking were comfortable temperature, quiet, the flexibility to change office furniture to suit new jobs, and a place to work without distractions.

Seventy percent of the office workers polled reported

What's Important to Office Workers?

Item	Workers Considering it to be "Very Important"
Good lighting	88%
A comfortable chair	73
Good circulation of air	70
The right temperature for you	69
Machines and reference materials within easy reach	69
The opportunity to stretch and move around during the day	67
A place to work when you need to concentrate without distractions	63
Enough space to move at your desk	57
Quiet	53
A window	40
A place where you can go to relax	38
The ability to change your office furniture as your job changes	24

Source: The Steelcase National Study of Office Environments, No. II: Comfort and Productivity in the Office of the '80s. ©1980 Steelcase Inc.

that they had personally complained about some aspect of office comfort. The biggest complaints were temperature (41 percent were either too hot, too cold, or otherwise discontent), space (22 percent were overcrowded or cramped), and physical environment (18 percent complained of noise, lighting, or cigarette smoke).

Enough statistics. The bottom line is that workers are well aware of the effects of their offices on their comfort and productivity. And a good many office workers aren't particularly pleased with their working environments — even in those offices with the latest in furnishings and modern technology. But it isn't simply a matter of keeping workers pleased that makes office design an issue worth discussing. Such "discomforts" as bad chairs or too many distractions or inadequate air conditioning may contribute to physical and psychological stress among workers. That stress, in addition to decreasing productivity and increasing absenteeism, can result in a wide variety of illnesses and ailments.

For example:

• Improperly designed chairs can cause varicose veins, bad backs, and other musculoskeletal disorders as well as contributing to psychological stress. Moreover, E.R. Tichauer, a professor of human factors at New York University, believes that a properly designed chair could add as much as 40 productive minutes to the working day of most people — that's about 21 extra productive days a year.[1]

• "Open" or "landscaped" offices, which have become commonplace in modern business facilities, may be cost-effective structures, but they may cost more than they save through reduced productivity resulting from too much noise, poor ventilation, and inappropriate designs — all of which may contribute to physical and psychological ailments.

• The rigidity of many office designs — even among the so-called "flexible" open offices — dictates rigidity in office procedures and worker behavior, often contributing to decreased job satisfaction and productivity and increased boredom and psychological stress.

Despite the concerns and complaints of workers, there seems to be insufficient concern among employers about the effects of office design on their workers' comfort and satisfaction. In the Harris poll, only 41 percent of the workers surveyed felt that their immediate supervisor was concerned about their comfort on the job; fewer than one worker in three felt that top executives were concerned. When the same question was asked of executives, 75 percent felt that they were sufficiently concerned about employee comfort.

Why the big discrepancy? Here's one possible answer: "There's a general feeling among bosses that if they provide attractive offices for their employees, they needn't worry about anything else," says a Chicago-based interior designer for several "Fortune 500" companies. "But you can be well-versed in 'space planning' or 'management efficiency' and know nothing about 'human factors' or 'environmental psychology.' "

The blame must be shared by office equipment manufacturers, who generally sell products such as computer terminals or furniture systems based on presumed efficiency and aesthetics without regard for their effects on the people who use them. Ironically, the equipment's shortcomings may substantially undermine the products' productivity claims. Manufacturers often aren't aware of these shortcomings, either — partly because worker comfort isn't a part of their consciousness, and partly because the effects of worker comfort haven't been fully studied or understood.

But enough is understood to know that there is an incredible lack of knowledge about workers' needs when it comes to the design of office environments.

FORM VS. FUNCTION

The modern office evolved out of the factories of the 1800s. With the industrial expansion that followed the Civil War came vast increases in industrial production, accompanied by similar increases in the paperwork needed to run the thriving new businesses. To accommodate this new adjunct to industrial production, small armies of clerks were organized into increasingly specialized departments. The large office began to resemble the factory, both in appearance and in function. Early offices relied upon the creation of superficial visual order — identical furniture and the precise alignment of desks to create the impression of corporate order.

The work flow itself was arranged in the fashion of the factory. By pooling clerical workers, for example, an executive could allow uniformity in salaries, supervision, record keeping, work standards, and environmental conditions. Even more important to the executive was that the importance of the individual clerk was decreased: If one was absent, work could be passed along to another worker without any loss of efficiency. Moreover, pooling allowed executives to isolate themselves from the noise of offices; an additional effect was to isolate bosses from all but the most superficial contact between themselves and their workers.[2]

Not much changed in the organization and design of offices for a number of years, although typewriters and adding machines were brought in during the early 1900s to "automate" many tasks that had been done manually. Women began to enter the office work force in large numbers around World War I, encouraged by eager employers who discovered that young women were willing to work for considerably less money than young men.

In the mid-1950s, something happened to help forge the link between office work and factory work. A management consulting team in Germany, the Quickborner Team, invented the "open office landscape." Its purpose was not interior design or decoration, but efficiency. The team had done extensive studies of the movement of paper through the office and began to plot those work flows on paper. They realized that offices would work best when their designs were based on the flow of materials and components, similar to the way that factories had been designed for years.

That was the beginning of the "open office," a subject that we'll return to in a moment. Suffice it to say that the modern office, like the modern factory, is designed around processes, not people. That alone wouldn't be so bad, particularly if the designs worked. But there are indications that they might not be working quite as well as expected — that we might, in fact, have brought into the office a number of the same problems that have long plagued the factory: psychological stress from routinized work and job dissatisfaction; pressures resulting from having to balance family life with a low-paid, dead-end job; and physical stress from poorly designed workstations that intended workers to be as interchangeable as paper clips.

Such problems are hidden beneath the aesthetic interior design of many modern office environments. Thanks to the magic of durable plastics, Formica, and upholstery, many cold, institutional office settings have been transformed into much more humane workplaces. If you open any architecture or interior design magazine, you are bound to find full-color glossy reproductions of such offices, many of which have received some award or another for design. Architects and designers like to give themselves awards and do so quite frequently — it makes them feel as if their creations are successful. And some of them are. But a lot of them aren't.

Despite the significant advances made in efficiency and design, architects and interior designers still have a long way to go in determining what constitutes a "good" design, as far as workers are concerned. Some researchers are surprised to find out that workers suddenly placed into an office considered to be "good design" don't necessarily prefer it to their previous (presumed "bad design") environments. This was demonstrated by Dr. Robert W. Marans, director of the Urban Environmental Research Program at the University of Michigan's College of Architecture. In 1979, Marans studied a recently built federal office building in Ann Arbor, Michigan. The Ann Arbor Federal Building was, like most newer federal buildings, attractively built, utilizing a variety of architectural innovations, from an indoor atrium to the landscaped office plans. The structure was given an award by the Michigan Society of Architects for design excellence, and a poll taken by Marans found that around three-fourths of the community thought the building was attractive.

Another architectural masterpiece, right? Wrong: In his survey, Marans also found numerous complaints by the workers in the Ann Arbor Federal Building. Around 75 percent — about the same percentage that approved of the building's design — were dissatisfied with it as a place to work. Nearly half rated it as a "fair" or "poor" workplace; one in three expressed dissatisfaction with individual workstations. The biggest complaints were typical of open offices: too much noise, poor air quality, too many distractions, and the inability to move around. Marans concluded that workers who were more content with their immediate work space were more content with the building as a whole.

Marans' revelations are part of a growing field called "post-occupancy evaluation," a process that seems light years behind its time. The idea is rather simple: After a building has been constructed and in use for a few years, to conduct an evaluation of how the building works — or doesn't. Simple as that sounds, it's a revolutionary concept among architects and designers, who are just beginning to discover that what works on paper doesn't always work in real life.

The few post-occupancy evaluations done of office spaces so far have shed some much-needed light on office design. One of the major users of the evaluations is the federal government, one of the world's biggest contractors of office space. For example, at the Norris Cotton Federal Office Building in Manchester, New Hampshire, the General Services Administration built in a number of energy-conservation measures, from solar energy to efficient lighting and heating systems. A comprehensive post-occupancy evaluation by the National Bureau of Standards revealed that the building rated favorably for lighting and acoustics, but unfavorably in terms of windows and temperature. The results have proved valuable to other building designers who have contemplated cutting costs through energy efficiency.

One reason that post-occupancy evaluations were so long in coming may be that office building designers were afraid to hear what building occupants thought about their work. In another post-occupancy evaluation conducted by the National Bureau of Standards — this one of the Richard H. Poff Courthouse and Federal Building in Roanoke, Virginia — employees listed three things they liked and disliked about the building. Their "likes" ranked in the following order: [3]
    1. Exterior design and appearance
    2. Nothing
    3. View
Not a terribly flattering appraisal, particularly since two of the three items had to do with the _outside_ of the building. The workers' "dislikes" included inadequate heating and air conditioning and too much noise, as well as dissatisfaction with amenities such as elevator service and parking facilities. Interior lighting was one area well-liked by most workers.

The purpose of the NBS evaluations was not just to critique office designs, however. As prototypes for the post-occupancy evaluation process, the NBS projects attempted to look at the *reasons* behind the problems and the successes. After their Roanoke study, NBS researchers tried to look backward into the design and construction processes to see who made inappropriate decisions and why they were made.

The answers offer a glimpse into some of the design problems that may be plaguing many other new buildings, and many of those buildings' occupants. For example, NBS concluded that the decisions that led to many of the Poff Building's major problems — including the ventilation system and the inadequate elevators — shared four characteristics:

1. They stressed costs above almost everything else;
2. They did not take into sufficient account the potential impact on building performance and user activities;
3. They were made without including the building's users in the decision process; and
4. They led to difficulties that might have been avoided if the building's users had been consulted in advance.

More about worker participation in the design of offices later on in this chapter.

Despite their obvious usefulness, post-occupancy evaluations of offices remain few and far between. And probably with good reason: With the exception of a few award-winning designs, most office buildings are still rather cold and dull. Corporations that pride themselves on their innovative approaches to problems suddenly lose that pioneering spirit when it comes to the problems faced every day by their own employees — opting, as GSA did, for cost considerations before anything else. Robert Propst, the design pioneer who developed the "Action Office" and other innovations for the Herman Miller Company, noted that "many people are ashamed of the way their work *looks,*" adding that "the ideal office of the design magazines was a fantasy that no one could live up to."[4] As another observer, Paul Goldberger, put it in *Saturday Review:* "Most corporate offices...are at best examples of efficiency only by accounting department standards, for they appear to have been built, above all, with an eye to the bottom line. Like public housing projects, they are designed to contain as many occupants as possible; to give each occupant an adequate amount of space, light, and air; and to be cheap to erect. In the view of most corporate executives, this is the definition of a building that 'works.'" What's worse, says Goldberger, is that "the executives who make the design decisions think their choices are good ones."[5]

Granted, most executives were not trained in human factors during their business schooling. They see their offices as so many desks and chairs, square feet and leases, paper and filing cabinets, fluorescent lights and machines. The office is a capital investment that must be streamlined to accommodate the ever-present bottom line. Nor are they helped along in this task by many office equipment and furnishings manufacturers or retailers, who tend to emphasize cost efficiency and the fact that "this is what everyone is using these days." Even professional designers, eager to please their clients with plush-pile carpeting and tasteful art, aren't knowledgeable about the "human factors" aspect of office environments — for example, the fact that word processing equipment may need subdued lighting and off-white walls to reduce glare into the eyes of users. Witness _Planning the New Office,_ a design-industry textbook, written by Michael Saphier, a well-known space consultant since the 1930s. The 230-page book deftly guides the budding designer through the bidding, buying, and building of office space — but gives virtually no information on human behavior or environmental psychology. There are six pages allocated to "personnel needs," but they deal mostly with the lunchroom and other amenities.

Offices designed for people tend to cost more, a clear disincentive for most money-conscious executives, who usually fail to recognize the link between environmental satisfaction and productivity increases — a link that many office workers have recognized for years. Unfortunately, the connection has yet to be made in most schools of architecture and interior design.

THE OPEN OFFICE

All of these failings are demonstrated neatly in the open office, a design that has virtually swept the country since the mid-1970s. The Steelcase study found that half of the nation's white-collar work force is now in open offices, and a survey conducted for the National Office Products Association concluded that such systems will outnumber traditional walled offices three to one by the end of the decade.

The open office of today is a direct descendant of the plan created by the Quickborner Team in the 1950s. In the typical open office, permanent walls give way to movable partitions, which typically stand five to six feet high. Within each workstation, desks, shelves, file cabinets, and even plants serve as space dividers between offices.

When the idea hit American offices, it hit hard. A big part of its attraction was that the open plan offered numerous advantages to the mushrooming office sector of the nation's economy: flexibility during a time of growth and change, increased control over design, improved work-flow efficiency, and improved cost efficiency. Manufacturers' brochures boast of the lower costs of open offices, as opposed to conventional walled ones, due primarily to tax incentives that allow movable furniture to be eligible for favorable tax treatment not afforded conventional offices. To the cost-conscious executive, it may all seem too good to be true.

Perhaps it is. Despite the still-growing popularity of the open office, there have been many problems associated with the designs. Not the least of those problems are too much noise, too many distractions, inadequate temperature control, and — ironically — inflexibility. That last complaint by workers came as something of a surprise to designers and manufacturers who had sold the designs to clients based upon their flexibility. It turned out that in many cases the personal work space in open-plan offices could not be manipulated as easily as in conventional offices. Workers in walled offices can rearrange them by moving bookcases, files, and desks. They often can turn lights on and off, open or close the blinds, perhaps even close a door. In open offices, however, furnishings usually serve as dividers between work spaces or dividers between offices and corridors and reception areas. One worker's file cabinet may be another worker's wall. When moved, it may alter the grand scheme. The "flexibility" promised by the manufacturers of open offices turned out to be for managers, who saved 75 percent or more of the cost of rearranging work space, in spite of one survey's finding that 75 percent of all white-collar workers never move their offices at all.

Workers themselves are not blind to the shortcomings. In an earlier Steelcase study, conducted in 1978, researchers asked workers to describe their feelings about their work spaces. Those in conventional walled offices tended to use words like "comfortable," "friendly," "impressive," and "home away from home," when describing their offices. Workers in open offices, however, more often singled out words like "functional," "modern," or "confining," indicating their offices' somewhat colder, albeit efficient, environment. When asked what they would most like to change about their work space, the two most common answers were "more privacy, to be separated from others or to have my own office" and "more personal space, a larger space."[6]

One thorough study of workers' attitudes toward open offices was conducted by Dr. Yvonne Clearwater, as part of her doctoral thesis at the University of California at Davis in 1979.[7] Clearwater, who is now an environmental psychologist in San Francisco, studied the reactions of 400 California state employees to their transition from conventional to open offices, one of the few comprehensive behavioral studies of such workers conducted to date.

Clearwater studied a large state agency that was in the process of consolidating its operations. The agency moved from locations scattered around Sacramento to a completely renovated building that had previously been a sprawling department store. During the course of the move, the employees left conventional walled offices for one massive room with few dividers, resembling the "bullpen" floor plan frequently encountered in newspapers, insurance companies, and stock brokerage houses, for example. Eventually, as movable screens were put up, the facility took on the characteristics of the "landscaped" office. Clearwater surveyed employee attitudes during all phases of the transition, making her study unique in its inclusion of all three major types of offices.

Clearwater concluded that open offices are not all that they're cracked up to be. "If one were to believe proponents' claims in popular design trade literature, one would expect that morale, communications, and productivity would rise considerably (and profitably) while window light continued to flow democratically through a more flexible workplace," she wrote. On the contrary, she said: "The fully landscaped office after three months was seen as less democratic. Every index of interpersonal and intra-organizational interaction and communications and friendship formations took serious turns for the worse....People felt insecure, unrelated, alienated, passive, and vulnerable."

Such feelings are easily understood when you look at the day-to-day working conditions of many workers, even those toiling for major corporations:

• In the headquarters of the Columbia Broadcasting System in New York — a 36-story corporate palace that has affectionately come to be known as "Black Rock" — secretaries are ranked from D (lowest) through G (executive). According to company policy, each is allowed no more than 60 square feet of working space, plus 15 square feet for files and machines; they sit at plastic-topped desks and use regulation equipment (such as the special CBS stapler) as dictated in the CBS administrative-services manual.[8]

• At a Blue Cross/Blue Shield office, also in Manhattan, Medicare investigators are required to clean their desks every night. Everyone must use the same type of file cabinet and waste-paper basket. No posters or photographs are allowed on the walls, and plants must be a certain height. Coats may not be placed in the back of desk chairs, but must be hung in a specially designed nook.[9]

• In a travel agency near Boston, clerks who take telephone reservations while working with video display terminals are allowed two ten-minute rest periods each day at predetermined times. If they happen to be on the phone taking a reservation during their break time, they simply miss it.

The efficiency of such standardized environments is what the open office is all about. After all, the whole idea was thought up by a German team to let bosses see at whose desks papers were bottlenecking, a situation that writer T George Harris called "a sort of mental nudist camp where nobody, not even executives, has any privacy." [10] But executives have considerably more options as to where they can escape to avoid the chaos.

Privacy — or, more precisely, lack of it — is a major problem with open offices. Actually, there are two kinds of privacy in the workplace: acoustical privacy (the ability to think and work without being disturbed by noise) and visual privacy (privacy from view of others). Of the two, acoustical privacy is more important to workers, according to the Steelcase study as well as work by other researchers. One study, by Dr. Jean Wineman, of Georgia Institute of Technology's College of Architecture, found that most people in an open office "reported being bothered by people passing their office who initiate conversation." Wineman found that despite claims by proponents of open office systems that open planning increases communication among workers, "My own work suggests that...these conversations are perceived as non-work related, while work-related conversations remain constant." [11] She also found that "although many workers were not bothered by their visibility to other workers, they felt that conversational privacy was lacking, especially for conversing with colleagues and clients, and for personal phone conversations." That finding was underscored by a previous survey of workers in open offices that found that 35 percent of workers in such offices were severely disturbed by noise and that only 20 percent were not bothered at all. [12] In still another study 54 percent of workers felt that their offices were sometimes so noisy that it was difficult to work. [13]

For more about the stress effects of noise in offices, see Chapter Six.

A CHAIR THAT FITS

Despite a significant amount of research on the subject, there have been precious few improvements in office chairs in recent years. Sure, there are some spiffy new models on the market, replete with ample upholstery and controls that move every which way, but you won't find these at the desks of many secretaries, clericals, or data processors. Instead, you'll find the basic "secretarial chair," which may or may not be appropriate for that particular person performing that particular job.

One of the big problems is that despite the dozens of studies of chairs and people, human factors experts — known variously by their many disciplines, including ergonomics, anthropomorphics, biomechanics, and industrial design — can't agree on what comprises an "appropriate" chair. For example, some researchers recommend that the seat of a work chair be parallel to the floor, while others recommend that it be tilted forward, and still others recommend that it be tilted back.

In fact, everyone might be right, since people come in a wide variety of shapes and sizes, and a variety of working and postural habits. The frustrations inherent in the "one-size-fits-all" approach to office furniture design are best demonstrated in a classic 1952 study performed by G.S. Daniels for the United States Air Force.

Daniels was charged with the mission of determining how many Air Force pilots would be considered "average" in terms of ten body measurements designed into Air Force clothing. He studied the measurements of 4,063 Air Force flyers to see how they compared with the "average" clothing they were wearing. He didn't even use an exact figure; in order to qualify as "average," an individual's measurements only had to be within 15 percent above or below the actual average measurement — a range of 30 percent. Here's what Daniels found: [14]

- Of 4,063 men, 1,055 were of "average" height.
- Of those 1,055 men, 302 were also of "average" chest circumference.
- Of those 302 men, 143 were also of "average" sleeve length.

- Of those 143 men, 73 were also of "average" crotch circumference.
- Of those 73 men, 28 were also of "average" torso circumference.
- Of those 28 men, 12 were also of "average" hip circumference.
- Of those 12 men, 6 were also of "average" neck circumference.
- Of those 6 men, 3 were also of "average" waist circumference.
- Of those 3 men, 2 were also of "average" thigh circumference.
- Of those 2 men, _none_ was also of "average" crotch length.

So much for "average" people. But that hasn't stopped furniture manufacturers from designing products for the "average" office worker.

There is little argument that poorly designed chairs can create serious physical problems. Back disorders are the number-one cause of absenteeism from work, and the second most prevalent disease in the United States (after sinus problems). They affect between 50 and 80 percent of the population and include complaints ranging from minor discomfort to major degeneration of the discs between vertebrae. Other problems include varicose veins, muscle cramps, and foot swelling, and there is some evidence that the arrangement of the body in various chairs can affect numerous muscles and nerves and interfere with the functioning of vital organs.[15] A poorly designed chair need not even be uncomfortable to cause such disorders; over prolonged periods, gradual damage can take place.

Human beings were not intended to sit. Our bodies were designed to walk — to follow our food, as our ancestors did for millions of evolutionary years. Chairs were alien to primitive cultures. It wasn't until the industrial revolution that we began to sit. Even in offices, chairs were not widely used until the turn of the century; accountants and other office workers either sat on high stools or stood. Today, we sit on chairs at home, school, in cars, at work, in buses — even on the beach. No one really knows exactly how much the typical person sits in a lifetime, but a conservative estimate would be that we spend at least a third of our time in that posture. By age 45, that amounts to 131,410 hours of sitting.

As with so many other aspects of the office environment, a great deal of study has been done in other countries — particularly Switzerland, Sweden, Germany, and Japan. Most of these countries have government-set standards about the design of chairs; no such standards exist in the United States.

Some American corporations have performed research on chair design too, of course. Herman Miller, Steelcase, and other major office equipment manufacturers have spent millions in research on new and improved chair designs. But because chairs remain a status symbol, the cream of this crop of new chairs ends up with executives and other top-level employees. Most workers get *assigned* a chair, as opposed to choosing one that fits into individual body dimensions and individual work habits. Many modern office chairs are adjustable to some degree, although not necessarily adjustable enough, leaving workers to choose one of a small variety of improper sitting positions. Still, the office chair remains perhaps the last component of the modern office that may still be manipulated at all by workers. Opening windows and adjusting lights and temperature are nearly impossible these days, and the nature of the work itself is rigid in many jobs too.

The problem with most chairs, ironically, is that they were not made for sitting for long periods. Prolonged sitting acts to restrict blood flow to the legs, which can lead to a number of circulation ailments, since blood flowing to the legs cannot easily return back up to the heart. A common ailment is varicose veins, resulting from excessive pooling of blood in the veins of the lower leg. Another is thrombophlebitis — the ailment made famous by Richard Nixon — which is an inflammation of the veins in the leg resulting from poor blood flow. These ailments also can result from sitting in a chair that is too high, requiring the legs to dangle, further cutting off blood flow.

Seats that are too low can cause problems as well. Such posture results in an awkward angle between the legs and the pelvis that puts pressure on the stomach, liver, and other abdominal organs. Over prolonged periods, this can result in severe pain.

Back problems from chairs result from insufficient support of the spine, both at the base and at the top. Most executive chairs are designed with full backs, but many "secretarial" chairs have extremely little back support: there is none at the base, and the small support that does exist often doesn't extend high enough to do any good. As one chair designer put it: "The secretary is seen in corporations as doing the most menial work, and the chair design reflects that kind of attitude." Some newer chair models have improved back supports, but these are more expensive than the less-supportive chairs.

Even the softness of the seat is important. Conventional wisdom has it that a soft seat is more comfortable and, therefore, better, but that is incorrect. A soft seat feels good only temporarily; eventually, the cushion will roll up around the sides of the buttocks, putting pressure on the hip joints. The seat's material also is important. Author and occupational health expert Dr. Jeanne M. Stellman recommends that it be of a porous material to allow body heat to dissipate — particularly important when wearing clothing made from synthetic materials, which tend to trap normal body heat and increase perspiration. Says Stellman: "Some experts even think that this daily build-up of heat and moisture can cause such medical problems as bladder infections or vaginitis."[16]

"You shouldn't even sit in the best-designed chair for more than 20 or 30 minutes at a stretch," says William Stumpf, a Winona, Minnesota, designer who has done some of the pioneering research in chair design as a consultant to the Herman Miller company. Stumpf says that part of the problem comes in the design process. "Some chairs are based around what I call the 'pilot syndrome,'" says Stumpf. "You assume that people are going to sit in one position all day, and the chair becomes a harness instead of a platform on which to behave in a variety of ways. I've done time-lapse studies of people sitting. It's like sleeping — you change positions constantly. I think the chair should support that change."

People sitting in office chairs tend to adopt one of three basic positions, says Stumpf. When thinking, reading, or talking on the telephone, one often sits back in the chair. Feet on top of the desk is another position — used to relieve the strain of prolonged sitting — although this isn't generally accepted office behavior for secretaries, clericals, and other relatively low-level employees, or for women of any level. Most of those people spend their time with feet tucked under the chair, body leaning forward into the work. It is in this "working" position that many problems occur, since most chairs are not designed to provide back support while leaning forward.

The inadequacies of chair design are evident even in executive chairs. The problem stems from the time-honored sexual biases that exist in many schools of design: secretarial chairs are designed for women, executive chairs are designed for men. Says industrial designer Don Albinson: "Most designers are men and the [executive] chairs they design are for men. They are too big for most women. An average women is less than 5'5". Women have longer legs and shorter waists. When a man tilts back, his weight is over the pivot point and the chair holds back. With a woman, the pivot plane is different, and she must work to hold the chair back in a tilt position. The woman sitting in a chair designed for men may tilt back, but the spring tension is difficult for her to overcome. If she releases too fast, it might just catapult her out of the chair."[17]

What constitutes a "good" chair? With the help of gadgets that measure blood flow, electrical potential of muscles during contraction, and the changes in angle between body segments, researchers have put together various recommendations. Here are some on which most agree: [18]

● The front of a work chair should be rounded off — often called a "scroll edge" or "waterfall cushion" — in order to avoid restricting blood flow in the underpart of the thighs.
● Support for the lumbar vertebrae (at the base of the spine) should be provided, helping the back to hold a slight forward arch. But while all researchers recommend lumbar support, opinions vary widely on exactly

where the backrest should be located, how high it should be, and of what contour.

• The seat cushion should have only light padding so that the buttocks can change pressure areas easily. If it is too soft, it puts pressure under the thighs, locks the hip bones upward, and pinches the underside of the socket joint.

• Backrests should be high enough to allow for relaxing, at least high enough to hit the lower few inches of the shoulder girdle, giving the arm a stable base against which to move.

• Just above the surface of the seat, the backrest should be either left open or so strongly concave that the ischium — the lowermost part of the hip bone, on which the body rests when sitting — can be rotated backward without hindrance. This also allows for air circulation.

• Seat height should be adjustable. Different researchers recommend ranges from 6 to 9½ inches of adjustability.

• Footrests should be provided for two reasons: for shorter people who must adjust their chairs too high in order to comfortably work on their desks; and for improving the angle of the foot when it is in a resting position.

• A headrest is suggested if the chair reclines. However, large rolls that push the head forward apparently are worse than nothing at all.

• There should be some mechanism for leaning the seat backward in order to rest strained back muscles. Movement back and forth, according to Dr. Juergen Kramer, encourages diffusion of essential nutrients to the viscous material in the intervertebral discs. Without those vital nutrients, the discs may degenerate, lose firmness, become flat, and in some cases bulge out, leading to various nerve disorders.

How to sit correctly. Even if you have an ideal office chair, it can all be for nothing if you don't use it right. Here are four suggestions on sitting:

• Keep your neck and back in as straight a line as possible with your spine. Bend forward from the hips, but don't arch your lower back.

• Use a footrest to relieve swayback. The idea is to have your knees higher than your hips.

• A few leg exercises at your chair during the day can minimize circulatory problems. For example: lift and lower your heels while keeping your toes on the floor; move your feet up and down while keeping your heels on the floor; and swing your legs back and forth at the knees. Even better, of course, is to walk around from time to time.

• Similarly, a few neck and shoulder exercises can relieve tension from prolonged sitting. For example: lift your shoulders to your ears and drop them down into a relaxed position; move your head up and down, side to side, and in a circular motion; and rotate your shoulders in a circular motion.

Additional relaxation and stretching exercises may be found in the Appendix.

THE OFFICE WORKER AS DESIGNER

There's a radical notion being knocked around progressive schools of architecture and design: Let office workers help design offices. It is shaking the very foundations of many dyed-in-the-wool professional architects and designers; for that reason alone, it may make a good deal of sense.

The concept is called "participatory design."

As the name implies, the idea is that users of office space be allowed to have a say in how it is designed. After all, who knows more than office workers about what works and what doesn't?

The few experiments so far indicate that participatory design works. In 1972, for example, Dr. Robert Sommer, a professor of environmental psychology at the University of California at Davis, along with three other design professionals, conducted a fascinating experiment for GSA. A federal agency was moving both its Seattle and Los Angeles offices at about the same time, providing an excellent laboratory for studying the effectiveness of participatory design.[19]

At the Seattle facility, workers were allowed to pick out their own furniture, choosing from various styles, colors, and materials. Rather than picking out items from

glossy catalogs, though, they were brought to a warehouse to inspect them firsthand. They were encouraged to
try them out — to sit in the chairs, stand at the tables,
write at the desks, etc. Group discussions were held so
that workers could discuss their needs with their co-
workers in the attempt to select office equipment that
would mesh with everyone's needs. "The employees were
good-natured during their visits to the warehouse, but
there were many expressions of skepticism that anything
would come of it," said Sommer, who headed the project.
"They had been so accustomed to having their work sta-
tions planned for them that the idea of individual choice
seemed alien."

At the Los Angeles facility, workers were treated to
the more traditional process of office designs selected for
them by interior designers. Several months after the two
groups moved into their respective buildings, a survey
was conducted of workers in the two facilities. The results:
The Seattle employees were more satisfied with their building than their counterparts in Los Angeles. Ironically, it
was the Los Angeles facility that was given numerous
awards by the American Institute of Architects; the Seattle
building received no such recognition. One member of the
AIA jury justified denying an award to the Seattle facility
on the basis of its "residential quality" and "lack of disci-
pline and control of the interiors" — precisely the qualities
that the Seattle employees liked most.

The entire cost of the planning process was $25,000,
excluding furnishings. Says Sommer: "It is clear that user
participation need not be expensive, and indeed may be
less expensive than other more traditional approaches."

Nevertheless, the notion that office workers should be
able to personalize the spaces in which they spend 40 or
more hours per week remains alien to the vast majority of
office designers. Sommer feels that such attitudes may
contribute to the apparent decline in morale and productivity in the nation's white-collar work force. In his book
Tight Spaces, he puts it this way:[20]

> Pleas for personalizing offices and work spaces are aca-
> demic and even precious until one sees the drab and im-
> personal conditions under which many people work. At

the offices of a large insurance company I found hundreds of clerk's desks in straight rows in a large open room with phones ringing, people scurrying about, and no one having any control over the thermal, acoustical, or visual environment....The quest for stimulating and attractive work places, the right to personalize one's own spaces and control temperature and illumination and noise are not academic issues to people who must spend eight hours a day in these settings. I don't feel it is necessary to "prove" that people in colorful offices will type more accurately, stay healthier, or buy more government bonds than people in drab offices. People should have the right to attractive and humane working conditions....This is a curious double standard. If an employee hangs up a poster by his desk, he is imposing his values and artistic tastes on the other employees, but if management paints all the walls in the building grey or institutional green, that is part of the natural order. We eventually tune them out and thereby become alienated from the very buildings in which we spend our daylight hours.

A footnote: Despite its apparent success in increasing employee satisfaction, the Seattle experiment in participatory design has never been repeated.

CHAPTER THREE

MORE THAN MEETS THE EYE

Office lighting is one of those things that always seems to fall by the wayside in discussions about the health of office workers. Sure, there are complaints: too bright, too dim, perhaps a slight feeling of irritation by the end of the day (although this could be attributed to a number of things). But how bad could the lights really be?

The lack of concern is shared by designers, executives, and facility managers. Lighting costs comprise a measly one-half of one percent of the office operating budget — not much to worry about, if you're an executive trying to trim costs. Few, if any, awards are given out for lighting, and a Very Important Client is not as likely to be impressed by innovative lighting as by sleek furniture or expensive art on the walls. Simply put, lighting just doesn't matter.

Or does it? We're just beginning to discover how wrong — and how unhealthy — that attitude is, for executives and managers as well as for secretaries and clericals. The nature of the office lighting under which workers spend around a fourth of their adult lives is suddenly becoming of interest to a growing number of scientists and other researchers who are coming to understand that bad light can make us unhealthy and good light can make us well.

But what exactly is "good" or "bad" light? Most people would be hard-pressed to answer that, and would find it even more difficult to evaluate their own office's lighting.

A typical educated guess might be that fluorescent lights are "bad," although no one would really be able to tell you why, or what kind of light was "good."

Yet despite this lack of knowledge about lighting by office workers, there is no lack of concern. In the comprehensive survey of office personnel conducted in 1980 by Louis Harris, "good lighting" was far and away the factor that most affected "personal comfort on the job." Eighty-five percent of the office workers and 83 percent of the executives polled responded that "good lighting" mattered "a great deal." Broken down by job description, 94 percent of the secretaries, 89 percent of the clericals, and 87 percent of the executives put lighting first in importance.[1]

For good reason: around 90 percent of the work performed in offices is visual.

But the Harris survey also found that only 66 percent of the respondents found their office's lighting to be "very comfortable," and 12 percent found it to be uncomfortable. One out of four workers thought that lighting conditions contributed to eyestrain. Broken down by job type, 34 percent of the clericals complained of eyestrain, compared with only 9 percent of the executives, managers, and supervisors, whose work typically is less visually intense than that of clericals and secretaries. The pollsters also found that 92 percent of the offices surveyed used fluorescent lighting as the primary light source.

The Harris Poll findings concurred with previous studies, such as the European work of A.C. Hardy in 1974, in which 900 workers rated the importance for their work of twelve environmental conditions. Good lighting ranked first in importance, followed by good ventilation, comfortable temperature, and plenty of space.[2]

Probably the most revealing statistic to come out of the Harris Poll was that nearly half of the executives sampled had never evaluated "lighting for office workers in terms of its effects on their comfort or productivity."

Granted, there hasn't been much good information available on lighting and its health effects on workers, despite a number of articles on the subject published in scientific journals dating back to the 1940s. Those few articles have provided a wealth of revelations about a subject

ing in front of a color television grew their roots up instead of down; mice raised under various types of fluorescents developed more fatal tumors, with the pink fluorescents turning out to be the most damaging; and a classroom of hyperactive children settled down when the standard fluorescent bulbs were replaced with a more healthful variety.[4]

Not all of these "findings" were well accepted, to say the least, and some were severely challenged, since they didn't stand up to the rigors of scientific analysis — which requires, for example, that the experiments be carefully controlled and repeatable. But whether precisely on target or not, Ott caused a number of people to stop and think about their lighting environments. Among those thinkers was a group of pedigreed scientists who agreed that Ott, while maybe less than "scientific," was on the right track.

Ott's principal point was a good one — that light, like food and water, is a nutrient that is vital to a healthy existence. As with food and water, insufficient light — or the wrong kinds — can cause ill effects. As this notion grew, and study of the health effects of lighting became more widespread, a new field of science was born: photobiology — the study of the effects of light on biological systems.

A LIGHT EXPLANATION

So, what constitutes "good light"? To understand the answer requires a brief understanding of the nature of "light" itself.

What is known as "visible light" is one small part of a spectrum of electromagnetic waves, known generally as "radiation." Radiation of varying wavelengths surrounds us constantly in the form of radio waves, microwaves, infrared radiation, ultraviolet light, gamma and x-rays — and visible light. The visible portion of the electromagnetic spectrum is a relatively tiny portion. If the entire electromagnetic spectrum were placed on a 100-yard football field, with each end resting on one goal line, the visible portion would stretch over less than one yard, even when combined with the invisible ultraviolet segment, which is another component of sunlight. Within this tiny span, there are a number of smaller segments, which we'll get to in a moment.

The sun, of course, is the principal source of light on our planet. Life evolved under sunlight — for plants and animals as well as for humans. Our eyes evolved biologically to sunlight and are entirely adapted to it. Only within the past century have we spent much time indoors under artificial light; today, we typically spend between 75 and 90 percent of our time under such conditions.

Sunlight beams down to earth a full spectrum of solar radiation, including ultraviolet light and visible light — that tiny "one-yard" portion of the electromagnetic spectrum. That segment can be broken down further into smaller segments: "far" ultraviolet, "middle" ultraviolet, "near" ultraviolet, and the visible colors, each comprising a unique segment of electromagnetic waves — violet, blue, green, yellow, orange, and red. All told, the normal human eye can discriminate more than ten million wavelengths.[5]

That full spectrum of visible radiation has become the basis of an increasing body of knowledge about the health effects of light. Research conducted around the world has concluded that environments containing "deprived-spectrum" lighting — light that does not contain the full range of colors and ultraviolet light found in sunlight — are not as healthy as those containing "full-spectrum" lighting.

As the Harris Poll found, cool-white fluorescent lighting is the illumination source in more than nine out of ten offices, with the rest relying primarily on incandescent (bulb) lighting, which also contains a deprived spectrum. There's no secret about the reasons for the popularity of fluorescents: they are extremely economical and energy efficient. The inside of a fluorescent bulb is covered with a powder-like phosphor material. When the light is turned on, electrodes at each end of the tube shoot electrons along the tube's length, usually around 60 times per second. The electrons pass through the krypton, argon, or neon gas contained in the tube, releasing energy, which strikes the tube walls. The result is that the phosphor material "fluoresces" and emits light.

Make no mistake: The fluorescent bulbs that are used in virtually every office were designed for efficiency, not for health purposes. Because our eyes are most sensitive to the yellow and green portions of the color spectrum, the phosphor contained in cool-white bulbs makes the light emitted high in yellow-green content, and contains little or no light from the remainder of the lighting spectrum — including very little ultraviolet light.

THE RIGHT LIGHT

For all of its importance, ultraviolet light is widely misunderstood. The fact that it can cause sunburn and skin cancer leads many people to believe ultraviolet light is harmful, but it's a known beneficial substance as well. The confusion lies in the fact that there are different kinds of ultraviolet rays, distinguished by the frequency and size of their electromagnetic waves. "Middle-ultraviolet" light rays — the ones that tan and burn — have the potential to cause cancer. "Far-ultraviolet" rays also are dangerous, but most are filtered out by the layer of ozone that surrounds the earth.

It is the "near-ultraviolet" rays contained in sunlight — and lacking in most artificial light — that perform a wide range of biological miracles. By the time it reaches the earth, sunlight contains about ten times more near-ultraviolet light than middle-ultraviolet light, although the exact ratio depends upon the time of year and the precise location on earth.

Simply put, near-ultraviolet light is essential for human well-being. It plays a key role in a number of vital physiological processes, from the formation of bones to the functioning of a dozen different organs and glands. Such revelations are not new; research dates back to 1945, when R.M. Allen and T.K. Cureton concluded that ultraviolet treatments resulted in a reduction of colds as well as an improvement in fitness.[6] During the 1950s, measured doses of near-ultraviolet light were found to improve work efficiency and to decrease fatigability.[7]

The Russians know well the benefits of ultraviolet light. A good deal of Russian research, which has received little attention in the United States, indicates that ultraviolet light helps in the prevention of disease; it reduces the incidence of colds, viral infections, and functional disorders of the nervous system, and helps to prevent black lung disease in coal miners. In fact, Russian coal miners and some other workers who spend long hours in artificially lighted environments are *required* to be given regular doses of ultraviolet light to aid in prevention of disease. So acutely aware are they of the healthful effects of full-spectrum lighting that official Soviet policy states, "If the human skin is not exposed to solar radiation (direct or scattered) for long periods of time, disturbances will occur in the physiological equilibrium of the human system."[8]

One group of Russian researchers found "a shorter reaction time to light and sound, a lower fatigability of the visual receptors and improved working capacity" for individuals receiving additional doses of ultraviolet light compared with those who did not. Other Russian research has documented that the body's tolerance to environmental pollutants is increased by full-spectrum light and that such light increases the effectiveness of immunization procedures.[9] The West German government, another European pacesetter, restricts the use of fluorescent lights in public buildings.

Light has several other important biological effects. Light falling on the surface of the skin causes tanning, of course, but it also is absorbed into the skin and is instrumental in the formation of vitamin D_3. Vitamin D is essential for the normal metabolism of calcium and inorganic phosphate in humans; a deficiency of the vitamin makes it difficult for these two minerals to be absorbed from foods into the body. In children, the resulting deficiency can stunt growth, bow legs, and cause other deformities. In both adults and children, it can cause bone pain and fractures.[10] During the industrial revolution, when an entire population moved indoors to work in factories, which, in turn, were belching vast quantities of smoke into the air, rickets became quite common in England. The disease — which stems from a vitamin D deficiency and is marked by bending and distortion of the bones, especially in infancy and childhood — resulted partly from a lack of sunlight, with smoke and smog putting up an umbrella against the healthy transmission of sunlight, reducing the body's synthesis of vitamin D.[11]

The synthesis of vitamin D is an important process among older people. For one thing, the elderly don't absorb calcium from foods as easily as younger people do. Vitamin D deficiencies among the elderly are well known, particularly among the institutionalized, since they often have very little exposure to sunlight. There is evidence that vitamin D deficiencies among the elderly may contribute to weakened bones and increase the likelihood of a bone fracture in the event of a fall.[12]

For similar reasons, the fluorescent-lighted environment could be a contributor to increased tooth decay, since another function of vitamin D involves stimulating the production of calcium for teeth. In fact, three researchers found in 1971 that hamsters exposed to full-spectrum fluorescent light simulating natural sunlight had only one-fifth as many cavities as animals exposed to conventional fluorescent light. The severity of the tooth decay was ten times greater under the cool-white light than under the full-spectrum light. Moreover, the development of the hamsters' male sex organs under the cool-white light was only one-fifth as much as under full-spectrum light.[13]

Vitamin D_2, which is similar to D_3 but not as effective, is added to milk and other foods, although its use is being sharply curtailed in Britain and other European countries because of evidence that it can be toxic in large amounts, leading to kidney damage, increased cholesterol, and other adverse conditions.

Some of the more pioneering work on the effects of ultraviolet light on the human body has been done by Dr. Richard J. Wurtman, director of the neuroendocrine laboratory at Massachusetts Institute of Technology, and Dr. Robert Neer, of Massachusetts General Hospital. In the early 1970s, they studied a group of elderly, apparently healthy men at the Chelsea Soldiers' Home in Boston. During the winter, the men were exposed to controlled amounts of ordinary fluorescent and incandescent (bulb) light. During that time, they were able to absorb only about 40 percent of the calcium they ingested.

Then, one group's lighting was changed to full-spectrum fluorescents for eight hours a day. While the first group's calcium absorption dropped about 25 percent, the full-spectrum group's absorption increased by 15 percent. Wurtman and Neer concluded that "properly designed indoor lighting environments could serve as an important public-health measure to prevent the undermineralization of bones among the elderly and others with limited access to natural sunlight."[14]

Another study, conducted at the Austrian Institute of Sportsmedicine, correlated full-spectrum lighting to improved physical fitness. The study was conducted over a three-year period, with groups of students undergoing regular physical education classes under full-spectrum and deprived-spectrum lighting. When a series of fitness tests were given, the full-spectrum group showed significant improvement of physical work capacity, decreased heart rate, and increased oxygen intake.[15]

The implications for office workers are clear. Since office work itself creates physical stressors that can cause a variety of physical ailments — bad backs from improper seating, for example, or muscle fatigue from improperly designed video display terminal workstations — the ailments may be made worse by the inadequate nature of most office lighting. In fact, it may be possible that full-spectrum lighting could act to keep bodies significantly stronger so that such physical problems could be avoided in some people. Of course, the lifestyle outside the office helps to determine exactly how much exercise and how much full-spectrum light a person gets. But during winter months and for a large number of relatively sedate office workers who don't spend much time outdoors, there are indications that full-spectrum office lighting could help to maintain good health.

Unfortunately, full-spectrum fluorescent lights are not readily available. Only one company in this country manufactures true full-spectrum bulbs simulating sunlight — the Duro-Test Corporation of North Bergen, New Jersey, which markets such bulbs under the name "Vita Lite" — although other lighting manufacturers claim to sell such products too. Duro-Test, unlike General Electric and the other major light bulb makers, doesn't sell its product in stores; Vita Lites are only available direct from the company.

Light has other important effects on human well-being. Information about light coming into the eye is relayed through the nervous system down the spinal cord and back up to the brain to affect the function of the pineal, a small but important gland located just above the eyes. The pineal, among other things, secretes melatonin, a hormone that plays a key role in the maturation of the ovaries. The pineal gland produces melatonin during the absence of light; therefore, melatonin production is highest at night. Light, entering the eye and reaching the pineal, stops production of melatonin.

Melatonin is needed to regulate your body's two main biological rhythms: "circadian" rhythms — 24-hour cycles that help the body know when to eat and rest; and reproductive rhythms that take place over the course of a year, such as a woman's four-week ovulation cycle. Studies by Dr. Alfred J. Lewy at the National Institute of Mental Health found that when melatonin production in animals is stopped, they refuse to mate, or don't grow antlers, or cease other normal seasonal functions.

There are some general suspicions that artificially lighted environments may interfere with these rhythms in humans, but they are largely unproven. The theory goes something like this: Since our inner "clocks" evolved in a world where we spent days under sunlight and nights in relative darkness, our modern environments, which are artificially lighted most of the time, may upset the normal rhythmic cycles. It is possible, for example, that the artificially lighted environments under which we spend the bulk of our days do not act as well as sunlight to shut off the melatonin production. The result may be premature sexual development; after all, the theory goes, aren't today's girls reaching sexual maturity faster than their grandmothers did? The answers are highly theoretical, and far from proven.

What has been proven is that the presence of ultraviolet light actually can improve work performance in offices. For example, a study performed in 1974 at Cornell University demonstrated that full-spectrum fluorescent light simulating sunlight can have a positive impact on an individual's well-being and abilities. The researchers examined two groups of students studying for four hours under two different fluorescent light sources; significantly better visual acuity and less physiological fatigue at the end of the work period were exhibited when the work space was illuminated with full-spectrum light rather than with conventional cool-white light. No significant differences between the groups had been found at the start of the period.[16]

There have been other problems associated with fluorescent lights. One big problem is the 60-times-per-second "flicker" in which the light appears to vibrate. The flicker may not be readily noticeable, although it may be perceived subconsciously. The flicker — which results from the speed with which electrodes cause the fluorescent bulb to glow — has been suspected of contributing to headaches, eyestrain, and fatigue, and may be a factor in spurring seizures in epileptics.[17] A more common effect is simple irritation. If daylight or incandescent light is added to the fluorescent environment, such problems diminish, but may not go away entirely. Some newer fluorescent fixtures are designed with a "lead-lag," so that one bulb flickers off while the other remains on, and vice versa, thus lessening the impact of the flicker; however, these fixtures are more expensive and not yet widely available.

A potentially more serious problem could be the ability of fluorescent lights to cause mutations in cells grown in a test tube. This evidence came out of a study conducted in 1977 at a molecular-pharmacology laboratory of the National Cancer Institute near Washington, D.C.[18]

In the experiment, hamster cells were exposed to ordinary fluorescent light from four cool-white bulbs made by Sylvania, a division of General Telephone & Electronic Corporation. The lights were placed in two desk lamps about three inches above the cell cultures for one to three hours. The exposed cells showed mutation rates several times greater than the unexposed cells. But making the link between hamster cells and office workers isn't all that simple. For one thing, workers' bodies are substantially hidden from the light by clothing. For another, the ham-

ster cells were kept three inches from the lights for a prolonged period — a bit closer than the distance between the
lights and most humans. But the study raised some new
questions about fluorescents, and similar results in tests
by at least six other researchers brought new credence to
John Ott's theories and to others who've long been maintaining that there's something not quite right about fluorescent light.

Some additional light was shed on the subject in 1979,
when researchers at the Food and Drug Administration's
Bureau of Radiological Health tested five commercially
available fluorescent bulbs. They concluded that the mutagenic effects came from sufficient intensities of specific ultraviolet wavelengths, and possibly "the interactions
among these wavelengths." Like the others, the FDA researchers concluded that a great deal of additional study
is needed.[19]

BRIGHT THINKING

Nothing discussed so far has had anything to do with
the *amount* of light that should be shed upon office
workers. Over the years, the "common wisdom" about how
much light is needed to do office work has gone full circle.
A century ago, before the common use of light bulbs, one
or two footcandles (an international measurement of illumination) was considered sufficient for reading. In the
1920s, the "Geneva Code of the International Congress on
Illumination" recommended five footcandles for proper
lighting. By the 1940s, as we found out that we could virtually light the night with cheap energy and modern technology, lighting engineers were claiming that the optimum level was 250 or more footcandles, with levels as
high as 500 footcandles being not unusual.

Then came the Arab oil embargo, the "energy crisis,"
and some new studies showing that we are perfectly capable of getting by with around 75 footcandles, or even 50,
depending upon the difficulty of the work, the size of the
reading material, and other variables. Later, lighting designers lowered those levels even more. Typical levels recommended for offices now are 50 footcandles for book-

keeping and typing, 40 footcandles for transcribing, 30 footcandles for filing and general correspondence, twenty footcandles for reception areas, and eight footcandles for entrances, halls, corridors, and other passageways.[20] Where video display terminals are used, ideal lighting levels are relatively low: around ten to twenty footcandles, according to one recommendation.[21]

(The above measurements also are commonly expressed as "lux" and as "lumen per square feet," two international measurements of illumination that have gradually replaced the footcandle. One footcandle is the equivalent of one lumen per square foot, or 10.76 lux. One lux equals one lumen per square meter, or 0.0926 footcandles.)

More recently, lighting engineers have begun to have some second thoughts about the lowered levels of lighting found in the energy-conscious office of the 1980s. For example, a study conducted by lighting engineers in 1979 at the Connecticut General Life Insurance Company attempted to "relate workers' lighting needs to their work performance and satisfaction, and to determine the cost-effectiveness of lighting." In the study, workers in a large insurance office performed normal tasks under three levels of illumination: 50, 100, and 150 footcandles. The researchers analyzed workers' evaluations and reactions to the work space and compared those evaluations to the workers' performance at the typical range of office tasks — reading handwritten copy, reading carbon copies, typing on forms, using microfiche, etc.[22]

The researchers found that workers preferred the brighter work space. Workers rated the 150-footcandle environment more than 40 percent higher than the 50-footcandle environment, and were more satisfied with eye comfort and stimulation. Similarly, there were significant improvements in worker performance and accuracy in the brighter work space: productivity improved 8 percent between 50 and 150 footcandles, and errors decreased by 18 percent. Finally, the researchers concluded that despite the tripling of energy costs between 50 and 150 footcandles, savings in increased productivity would amount to more than $2,000 a year per worker.

But too-bright lights may pose problems, as light bounces off reading material — particularly the glossy paper of magazines and some books — into the eyes. Bright, uniform ceiling light also bounces off the ceiling and walls and into workers' eyes. Over prolonged periods, the intense light can blur objects and cause the eye's retina to lose the precise adjustment it needs for clear vision.

Ultimately, lighting needs are highly individualized, depending upon the type of work being done and an individual's eyesight. The research on lighting requirements often is done at universities using college students with good vision as the norm.[23] But when eyes get older, they need more light; a twenty-year-old's lighting needs may be totally inappropriate for a 50-year-old office worker.

What makes sense, then, is "task" lighting — a notion that became popular in the mid-1970s with the advent of the "open" or "landscaped" office, but which is applicable to any office environment. As with many other aspects of the modern office, the flexibility that allows workers to meet their own individual needs often creates the most satisfaction and the least amount of stress for all involved.

LIGHT AND COLOR

Color is another factor in the quality of lighting, although its effects are largely psychological — and somewhat controversial. "White" light, after all, is made up of colors, and in fluorescent lights, the specific color given off depends upon the types of phosphors used. The standard "cool-white" lamp is high in yellow and green; "warm-white" lamps contain somewhat more of the red-orange phosphors. Incandescent light is extremely high in red-orange output, since its light is produced by the heating of the filament inside a bulb. The light given off by full-spectrum fluorescents, a balanced light output that simulates sunlight, appears to be somewhat bluish, the same pale blue cast you see when you look outside.

Such color differences may seem to matter only to personal preference, but they can affect performance. It is well known that colors have an effect on our physical and psychological well-being. "Seeing red," "feeling blue," and "in the pink" may just be three colloquial expressions, but they have some basis in color psychology. Red, for example, is associated with intensity and rage; blue gives an impression of gloom and fearfulness; pink suggests youth, gentility, affection.

Such interpretations come from Faber Birren, considered by many to be the foremost authority on the effects of color on behavior. His many respected books and essays — *Color and Human Response,* published in 1978, is his best known — have revealed a great deal of information about the effects of colors on our lives. Among his conclusions:[24]

- Red tends to raise blood pressure, pulse rate, respiration, and perspiration. It also helps to increase tension.
- Blue tends to have a reverse effect, lowering blood pressure and pulse rate, decreasing perspiration and brain waves.
- Green tends to be more or less neutral.
- Orange and yellow create similar reactions as red, but less pronounced.
- Reaction to purple and violet is similar to that of blue.

Environmental colors, of course, come largely from colors of walls, furniture, and other surroundings, but the color of lighting can affect the way that walls and furniture appear before our eyes.

That the color of light can create unpleasant effects on humans has been shown in offices and schools where high-pressure sodium vapor lights have been used. Sodium vapor lights have become increasingly popular among lighting designers in recent years due to their high energy efficiency. Unfortunately, they emit a light that is extremely high in yellow content, a factor that can make sodium vapor-lighted environments extremely unpleasant. One reason is that sodium vapor light distorts color rendition, which can result in disorientation and in headaches, dizziness, nausea, and fatigue. In an elementary school in Connecticut, for example, young children and their teachers experienced such symptoms as a result of sodium vapor lights. When the lights were replaced — at a cost of $30,000 — the symptoms went away.[25]

Sodium vapor lights aren't very popular among office workers either. Dr. Jean D. Wineman, of Georgia Institute of Technology, evaluated 30 workers who were moved from an office space illuminated with traditional fluorescent lights into a space illuminated with high-pressure sodium lights. Immediately before and after the move, workers generally were satisfied with the light. But not long following the move, complaints concerning shadows, low overall levels of light, and lighting contrasts increased. Wineman concluded that "people require higher levels of light to reach a given level of satisfaction, if they feel a light source gives poor color rendition."[26] Ironically, Wineman's finding belies the improved energy efficiency claims made by the manufacturers of sodium vapor lights.

Wineman's study is not the first to conclude that the quality of lighting affects the *perceived* brightness (in other words, the better the quality of the light, the brighter it seems to be, even if the illumination levels are actually lower). Not surprisingly, natural lighting through windows is the most desirable. In her research, Wineman cites studies suggesting that "people whose office locations are closer to the windows rate the quality of lighting more highly than people located farther from windows." Yet, lighting levels near windows vary considerably more than in other parts of the office, due to the light changes during the course of a day. It's the *quality* of the light that makes it more satisfying.

THE BOTTOM LINE

How much do factors like color satisfaction and lighting levels really have to do with office worker health? The answer to that depends upon what one considers to be "health." A company executive is likely to pooh-pooh the notion that office lighting can make workers sick. After all, the executive came up through the ranks of the office, working in conditions that were far less cushy and considerably less bright than in the modern office. And, since the executive hasn't had any ill effects, why should anyone else?

The argument may seem convincing, but it holds no water. For one thing, the office of the past — even of five years ago — is different from the office of today. Physiological and psychological stress levels may be higher in the modern office due to a variety of pollutants, design deficiencies, the increasingly routinized nature of office work, and other factors. There's a case to be made that lighting can contribute to that stress if it is too bright or too dim, if it creates glare, if its color is even slightly distasteful, or if it contributes to ill health.

The "bottom line" is this: In terms of actual dollars spent, lighting costs typically are less than 1 percent of office operation costs, and employee costs are more than 80 percent. But the lighting costs actually may be significantly more, if lights are contributing to decreased productivity and increased absenteeism. As was shown in the Connecticut General study, there is a "positive relationship between lighting conditions in the work space and the degree of worker satisfaction and productivity." That study also found that a reduction of even one-half of 1 percent in employee performance could cost much more than the price of an improved lighting environment.

If employers and office designers could look past price tags and simple solutions, office workers might be happier, healthier, and more productive. When that's the case, everybody wins.

CHAPTER FOUR

TERMINAL ILLNESSES

With the introduction of the integrated circuit into the workplace during the 1970s, computer terminals took a firm hold in businesses large and small. As computer sizes and costs diminished, and simplicity and capabilities grew, the long-awaited "office of the future" began to come to fruition in a big way.

In the next few years, computerization will link most major office machines into one vast network: Photocopiers will not merely make copies, they will send them electronically to specified destinations over telephone lines or via satellite transmissions; the copies will be printed at or near their recipients' desks on high-speed printers or will appear on computer screens; permanent copies may be made on microform or stored in computers for later reference. Information flows will be accelerated exponentially, with time lags measured in minutes instead of days.

The human link to all of this, of course, is through the computer's video display terminal (VDT), known also as a video display unit (VDU) or a cathode ray tube (CRT). It is through this television-like screen — familiar to anyone who's used a 24-hour electronic banking terminal — that users enter and retrieve information. There are somewhere between seven and ten million people working on VDTs in the United States, plus a similar number in other countries. Those figures are expected to grow three to four times by the end of the decade.

To put it bluntly, most VDTs are bad news. A wide

range of problems have been associated with VDT use, due partly to the "ergonomics" (design) of the machines, and partly to the way in which they are used. In the few short years VDTs have been in widespread use, they have been found to cause a number of serious problems to users: Moderate-to-heavy use of VDTs frequently leads to eye-strain, loss of visual acuity, changes in color perception, back and neck pain, stomachaches, and nausea, to name just a few of the ailments reported.

That's just for starters. In addition to the physical stress produced by VDTs, the devices have been associated with levels of psychological stress substantial enough to contribute to a further array of ailments ranging from headaches to heart attacks. Moreover, VDTs — and the other components of the modern electronic office — may produce potentially harmful levels of microwave and other types of radiation; more on that in the following chapter. And despite the optimistic projections of future growth of VDT use, researchers are just beginning to raise questions about what the long-term effects of VDTs will be.

VDT operators are by no means blind to the problems. A good many operators are acutely aware of them, as indicated by the concern of labor unions and other organizations surrounding their use. In January 1980, for example, the New York Committee for Occupational Safety and Health (NYCOSH) conducted a conference "directed solely at clerical workers" who have suffered adverse health effects from VDTs. Nearly 350 people showed up, with others being turned away for lack of room. At the conference, workers listened to experts and aired their litany of complaints against video display terminals.[1]

To be sure, there is little wrong with the new technology in terms of its ability to increase office efficiency and — potentially — to make work life easier both for workers and their employers. Business computers are extremely powerful tools with an increasing number of valuable applications. In the relatively few short years they have been in use, VDTs have become indispensable parts of the publishing, insurance, communications, and banking industries, and are used widely in most other industries as well. VDTs are gradually appearing in homes — marketed as "personal computers" — and they are expected to become a principal medium for communications in coming years. Even the most vociferous opponents of office automation base their opposition not on the mere existence of the technology, but on its effects on the office work force.

Basically, a video display terminal operates much like a television set. The difference is that the images that appear on the screen originate from a computer instead of from a TV camera. A VDT contains a source of electrons and a phosphor-coated screen within a specially designed vacuum tube. Under high voltage, electrons are emitted by the electron gun, or cathode, and accelerated toward the screen. The gun scans the screen at a predetermined rate — say, 50 times per second — and projects electrons according to an electronic signal. When the electrons interact with the phosphor coating of the screen, visible radiation — light — is produced and an image is formed. This is referred to as a "raster scan" process; "rasters" are the horizontal lines you can see on a television screen if you look closely enough. On a VDT, the rasters form the letters on the screen; a capital "M" might be seven rasters high, for example.The more rasters per character, the sharper the screen image.

The problems associated with video display terminals are being studied at an increasingly frantic pace by government agencies, unions, and universities around the world. More than two dozen major studies have been performed since 1975, revealing a wealth of information about the effects of this new technology. Most of the earliest and most thorough studies were done outside the United States, primarily in European countries like Sweden, Austria, and West Germany, which have aggressive government-sponsored programs examining a wide range of occupational health and safety issues. One of the earliest pioneers in this still-emerging field of technology health science is Dr. Olov Östberg, whose work for Sweden's National Board of Occupational Safety and Health during the early 1970s remains the most comprehensive look at the problems associated with VDTs.

In a 1975 article in *The International Journal of Occupational Health and Safety,* Östberg outlined some of the disturbing problems associated with VDTs. The article, he said, was aimed at "encouraging manufacturers and users of modern office equipment to pay closer attention to early signs of nuisance to operators caused by lack of ergonomics considerations — otherwise this nuisance will soon be manifested as occupational illness."[2] Sadly, most manufacturers and users failed to heed Östberg's warning, and computer use has grown astronomically.

One of the most thorough surveys of such problems was conducted in 1979 by the National Institute for Occupational Safety and Health (NIOSH) at four newspaper offices and a major insurance company in the San Francisco area. The study was instigated at the request of a coalition of five international unions — Communication Workers of America, the Newspaper Guild, Office and Professional Employees International Union, Graphic Arts International Union, and Transport Workers Union of America — and by nineteen local unions and two regional councils. In their letter to NIOSH, the self-proclaimed "VDT Coalition" expressed concerns that workers did not have the necessary information about the effects of VDTs to conduct informed and fair collective bargaining with employers who were introducing the technology into the workplace at a rapid rate. The coalition requested that NIOSH "conduct an in-depth study that can answer the variety of questions raised by users of video display terminals."

In one aspect of the study, NIOSH surveyed 250 VDT operators and 150 control subjects who did similar work not involving VDTs. The work being done by these 400 individuals included the typical range of office work: data entry and retrieval, word processing, writing, editing, and telephone sales. Both clericals and "professionals" (mostly reporters, editors, and copy editors) were included in the survey.[3] The health problems identified are summarized in the table on the following page.

It's difficult to neatly categorize all these various problems by their causes, since causes are often coupled with environmental factors and the nature of the work itself. But for matters of simplicity, the problems of VDTs may be divided into three types: eye problems, physical stress, and psychological stress.

Health Complaints of VDT Users

Complaint	VDT Users	Non-VDT Users
Eyestrain	91%	60%
Painful/stiff neck or shoulders	81	55
Burning eyes	80	44
Irritability	80	63
Back pain	78	56
Fatigue	74	57
Irritated eyes	74	47
Blurred vision	71	35
Sore shoulder	70	38
Painful/stiff arms or legs	62	35
Neck pressure	57	34
Skin rash	57	31
Neck pain into shoulder	56	19
Stomach pains	51	35
Nervous	50	31
Swollen muscles and joints	50	25
Hand cramps	49	16
Numbness	47	18
Stiff/sore wrists	47	7
Change in color perception	40	9
Pain down arm	37	20
Fainting	36	17
Loss of strength in hands/arms	36	14
Loss of feeling in fingers/wrists	33	11

Source: National Institute for Occupational Safety and Health, "An Investigation of Health Complaints and Job Stress in Video Display Operators," 1980.

EYE PROBLEMS

As the data in the accompanying table indicate, complaints of eye problems are widespread among users of VDTs. Such general complaints as strain, burning eyes, and blurred vision are common among office workers generally — including managers and executives — but are often twice as high among those who use VDTs for even a few hours a day. In 1979, two Swedish researchers found that at one insurance company, 84 percent of those who experienced visual strain in their daily work were affected after only 90 minutes of VDT work.[4] There is no conclusive evidence that VDTs contribute to any permanent eye damage (although some VDT users have reported frequent refitting in prescription lenses), but even as temporary phenomena, such discomforts can severely affect an individual's ability to be productive in the workplace and to perform other non-work-related visual tasks comfortably, including reading, driving, and watching television. The problem of VDT-generated cataracts, a burning issue among users of VDTs, is discussed in the next chapter.

A brief explanation of how the eye focuses on an object may be helpful to understand the nature of VDT-related visual problems.

Much like a camera, the eye has two kinds of adjustment mechanisms: variable focus and variable light. Changes in the amount of light that enters the eye are made by automatically regulating the size of the pupil. Changes in the point upon which the eyes focus are made automatically by the brain's command to adjust the set of ring-like ciliary muscles that surround the lens. A circle of tiny, spider-web-like fibers, the zonular fibers, stretch from the ciliary muscles to the lens and hold it in place. At the command of a special nerve coming from the brain, the contraction of the ciliary muscles tightens or loosens the zonular fibers. The pull, transmitted to the lens of the eye, changes its shape just enough to refocus the eye for a particular distance. This act of focusing is called "accommodation." In addition, exterior eye muscles are called into action — in all, some 22 different interior and exterior eye muscles are utilized during accommodation.[5]

When your eyes are relaxed — that is, not looking at anything in particular — the ciliary muscles are naturally focused on distant objects "at infinity." Most everyone recognizes this phenomenon as "staring off into space." When you focus on a close object, the muscles contract so that the eyeballs can turn inward, which creates tension in the ciliary muscles. The extreme example of this is the pain you feel when you try to look at the end of your nose for a prolonged period. If the muscles must remain contracted for long periods of time, they get tired — what's known to most of us as "eye fatigue." Continued tension in the ciliary muscles can cause headaches, eye discomfort, and — ultimately — "double vision," resulting from loss of coordination between the two sets of ciliary muscles.

These problems are somewhat more troublesome for older people, who are often affected with "presbyopia" (*presby* = old, *opia* = eyes), a natural part of the aging process. The older person's eyes lose pliability of the lens, making the accommodation process more difficult. Moreover, pupils tend to decrease in size during later years, and other parts of the eye become less effective, making older people more susceptible to glare and to other less-than-ideal lighting conditions.

Having understood the general nature of "eyestrain," it is easy to see how prolonged staring at a VDT that is approximately ten to eighteen inches away can strain eye muscles. But that is not the only factor that comes into play to create eye problems.

Lighting. One simple notion that seems to have eluded the majority of office architects and designers is that the lighting conditions needed for VDT work are far different from those needed for filing, typewriting, using adding machines, and performing other non-VDT-related work, including using computers that utilize punch cards, printouts, and other "hard-copy" formats. In such environments, workers need lighting that is sufficiently bright to illuminate the tasks. But with VDT work, considerably *less* light is needed in order to maximize contrast of the words on the VDT screen and to minimize glare on the screen resulting from overhead lighting; individual "task" lighting may be needed to provide enough light to read printed copy.

This all seems simple enough, of course, but if you visit almost any office that contains computers using VDTs, you'll find VDT operators sitting side by side with typists and file clerks, all working under the same lighting conditions — usually banks of "cool-white" or "warm-white" fluorescent lights. The result is twofold: VDT screens not only don't have optimum contrast due to excessive lighting, but must compete with glaring lights, which bounce off the screen and into operators' eyes. Such conditions not only further contribute to eyestrain, eye fatigue, and other eye problems, but require operators to adjust their posture in an attempt to eliminate or minimize the glare, which in turn contributes to the variety of physical problems revealed in the NIOSH survey. (More on physical problems in a moment.) And to top it all off, the inability to properly view one's work is another contributor to psychological stress. (More on that in a moment too.)

Windows. Excessive lighting isn't the only source of glare. Large, bright windows — aesthetically desirable to virtually every office worker — are another source, unless they are sufficiently covered with shades or curtains. Unfortunately, VDT operation often takes place in large, partitioned "open offices," in which windows often are (and should be) available for all workers in the area.

Walls. A third source of glare are brightly colored walls, ceilings, desks, and even the computer keyboard. "Many people's idea of computer technology is that it is nice and shiny and clean and white," says Dr. Jeanne M. Stellman, director of the Women's Occupational Health Research Center at Columbia University and author of *Women's Work, Women's Health* and *Work is Dangerous to Your Health,* two excellent references on occupational health and safety. "And when you look at display terminals, they're almost always set up on a shiny white desk, with a nice white Formica finish." Because the eye's pupil automatically adjusts to accommodate the *total* amount of light entering the eyes, a bright background will cause the pupils to contract (become smaller), making it difficult to read the relatively dim light on the VDT screen. White isn't the only color that can cause problems; yellow, orange, and other bright wall colors can have a similar effect, unless they are of matte (light-absorbent) material. Ironically, such colors are the ones most common to the open-office partitions manufactured for modern offices.

Image size and sharpness. Another source of eye problems is the size of the letters on the VDT screen. Less-expensive computer systems often come with smaller screens, which usually display smaller characters in order to maximize the amount of information that can be displayed on the screen at any one time. Smaller character size frequently requires the operator to move closer to the screen — which can result in physical stress after a prolonged period — or to strain the eyes further in an attempt to read the screen from a distance. To make matters worse, some machines' letters do not appear sharp and clear, creating additional eyestrain, particularly for older workers.

Flicker. Still another source of problems is inherent in the nature of the cathode ray tube used in virtually all VDTs. As previously described, the images that appear on a VDT screen result from an electron beam that sweeps horizontally across the inside of the screen. The beam sweeps the screen from top to bottom; after the bottom line is swept, the beam returns to the top and the sweep process repeats. The number of times per second that this takes place is called the "refresh rate."

If the refresh rate is sufficient (about 65 flashes per second or more), the images on the VDT screen will appear to be steady; if not, they may appear to "flicker." The flicker, even if perceived only on a subconscious level, can contribute to eyestrain as well as to psychological stress. But most cathode ray tubes — including ordinary television sets that are utilized as the reading devices on some computer systems — operate at less than 65 flashes per second. As a result, other factors such as size and brightness of images influence a user's ability to perceive the flicker. Some VDTs that flicker when used in brightly lighted offices will not appear to flicker when room lighting is lowered considerably and there is a corresponding lowering of the VDT's brightness setting.[6]

Machine maintenance. Visual problems can result from a lack of proper VDT maintenance. Images on improperly maintained VDTs, for example, are not as sharp as on those that are regularly inspected. Usually, degradation of screen images is so gradual that VDT operators do not notice it — although they suffer the effects of a less-than-sharp screen anyway.

Dirty screens are another problem. A former reporter at the *Washington Star* newspaper in Washington, D.C., which has tussled with two trouble-plagued computer systems since 1975, recalled the frustration he and other reporters and editors faced, a frustration echoed by office workers in offices around the country: "The system was really hell. The biggest problem was that they never cleaned the screens. I don't understand how some people saw through them. I was always calling the maintenance supervisor to get him to clean the machine, but he never came often enough. At one point, to get his attention, I took the cover off of the terminal and put it over my head and went up and talked to him through the dirty screen. Then he listened to me. His comment was, 'Who taught you how to do that? You're going to get electrocuted and screw up the whole system!' That's what he was worried about — that I might screw up the system."

PHYSICAL STRESS

When the effects of VDTs in the workplace were first examined, Olov Östberg and other researchers immediately discovered special problems associated with VDT use by older workers. But subsequent studies found that even younger workers faced difficult physical demands from VDT use not previously encountered in other office tasks. For example, Östberg and Ewa Gunnarsson studied a group of relatively young Scandinavian airline reservation clerks whose jobs involved intensive VDT work. Nearly two-thirds reported some form of frequent muscular discomfort; three-fourths complained of frequent visual problems as well.[7]

It's difficult to separate some of the physical problems from the eye problems. As we previously learned, glare on VDT screens forces users to adapt their postures to compensate for the reading difficulty. This and other problems often result from the inflexibility of many computer terminals: screens aren't adjustable, keyboards cannot be located to the most comfortable position, and the brightness and contrast of the images on the screen can't be altered.

One classic example of the problems associated with inflexibility comes from VDT operators who wear glasses. Normal reading glasses are designed to be used with a twelve-to-fifteen inch distance between the eyes and the reading material. When VDT screens can't be moved back or forward, nearsighted and farsighted operators are often forced to lean forward or backward to compensate. In 1976, a Swedish researcher named Carlsoo set out to find out why 51 percent of VDT workers in one office reported neck pains and 60 percent complained of back pains. The research involved making electromyographic (EMG) studies of nerve activity. The conclusion was that the back pains resulted from awkward working postures.[8]

The problems may be even worse for those who wear bifocals. Only a few VDT manufacturers design screens that can be adjusted up or down so that operators need not tilt their heads back in order to read from the bottom (reading portion) of their glasses. Ideally, the machine, its desk, and the operator's chair should be designed so that the user looks slightly down onto the screen. There also are indications that VDT work should not be done by those wearing contact lenses; the decrease in blinking while staring at VDT screens is suspected of causing a drying of the eyes, often resulting in severe discomfort.

But machines, desks, chairs, and the rest of the environment often are designed more for efficiency of space planning and cost competitiveness than for worker comfort. Modular furniture units with neatly built-in computer terminals and related equipment make moving day considerably less painful for office designers and managers, but they are somewhat more painful for computer operators who must adjust their posture and physical actions to accommodate the equipment, instead of the other way around. A good many of the top manufacturers of "state-of-the-art" business technology design products based upon their convenience and efficiency — "productivity-increasing devices," as they are termed in manufacturers' ads — despite the fact that these designs often are, in reality, inconvenient for users, substantially *decreasing* their work efficiency.

Another example is the design of computer keyboards. They also should be flexible to meet the varying needs of each user. The 15 percent of the population that is left-handed, for example, has different requirements for keyboard placement than the right-handed users. Operators must compensate for inflexible keyboard design by adjusting their posture, as they did to compensate for rigid lighting and screen designs. The frequent result, as the NIOSH survey found, is the disturbing rate of "painful or stiff neck or shoulders . . . back pain . . . sore shoulders . . . painful or stiff arms or legs . . . neck pressure . . . hand cramps," and other physical ailments experienced by VDT users.

Chairs, of course, are another crucial piece of this puzzle, since they in large part dictate sitting posture and the distance between the VDT and the operator. As described in Chapter Two, chairs should be adjustable in height as well as in the angle of the backrest, to allow for the optimal sitting position.

The general aches and pains listed in the NIOSH data aren't the only ill effects suffered by office workers as a result of poorly designed VDT workstations. Headaches and overall fatigue are common responses to the physical stress, as is increased difficulty in performing work duties efficiently. A group of Japanese researchers found that, along with the localized fatigue present in the arms and hands of some office workers, some VDT users experienced decreased grasping power and decreased speed and pressure of key strokes.[9]

PSYCHOLOGICAL STRESS

As stated previously, it's difficult to separate the psychological stress of working with VDTs from the physical stress — or even from the visual problems. But a number of additional factors come into play that help to make VDT-related work among the most stressful in our modern society.

In the NIOSH survey of VDT workers in California, researchers found "higher levels of job stress than have ever been observed on assembly lines," according to Dr.

Michael Smith, a NIOSH psychologist involved in the study. "It was just a shock to us. If these levels are found in other facilities that we are presently looking at, they are going to have a tremendous impact on productivity. There's no question about it: I think in the long run, these things are going to be counterproductive."

Shocking though this may be, Smith's findings are nothing new. Since the advent of computerization in offices, workers have been confronted with a laundry list of psychological stressors: compartmentalization of secretarial and clerical jobs, with tasks being broken down into smaller and more monotonous components of larger tasks; job speed and processes being dictated by computers, which require that specific functions be done in specific order, at predetermined speeds, without regard to individual preferences or abilities; pressures resulting from being watched over by supervisors who can measure keystrokes, input, mistakes, time off, and other things; fear that automation will put them out of work altogether.

The list goes on. A few years ago, such factors led to worker rebellions against automation in some offices. Now, most office workers recognize the inevitability of the new technology, so frustrations often are not as apparent. "Opposition to computers is usually kind of veiled or disguised under more general complaints about eyestrain, headaches, and physical discomforts often associated with VDTs," says Dr. Michael Colligan, another NIOSH psychologist. "But if you talk with the workers awhile, major concerns begin to surface."

"The computers are designed on the basis of how fast they can operate and not on the capabilities of the human operator who is putting information into the system," says Smith. "The difficulty comes when you have workload and work pacing that are related to the machine instead of the human. That puts a tremendous load on the operator. At the same time, the system can monitor a hell of a lot better than a supervisor can. This monitoring, in our studies, is shown to be a very significant factor. People feel that they are being watched continuously. They become paranoid.

"The supervisor gets continuous feedback from the machinery and runs back to the person every half hour and says, 'You're not as fast as you were yesterday. You've made more errors than you did yesterday.' They're monitoring strokes per minute, error rates, and when you sign off the tube to go to the potty. It has taken away any possible flexibility that was there before."

Smith's findings have been corroborated by other researchers, who have found that physical problems and psychological problems tend to feed off of each other. For example, Swedish researchers Ewa Gunnarsson and Inger Soderberg studied complaints of eyestrain by VDT operators at the Swedish Telecommunications Administration, and concluded that "visual strain was more frequently observed among operators whose work was highly structured, inflexible, and done under conditions of stress."[10] In other words, it appears that while some researchers have found that visual problems lead to psychological stress, others have found that a stressful environment can exacerbate visual and other physical problems.

But the physical stressors alone aren't to blame. A big factor is the nature of the work performed on VDTs. The essence of computers in the modern office is that they allow businesses to handle much more business, faster and more efficiently than with the traditional "paper-pushing" procedures. Among other things, computers allow an increased work- or data-handling capacity per employee which generally decreases the number of skills used per employee. Secretaries who once handled a letter from dictation to transcription to final copy to mailing may find themselves simply transcribing notes — or assembling preprogrammed paragraphs — onto VDTs for six or seven hours per day, while the other tasks are handled by other individuals on the word-processing assembly line. Data-processing clerks who once turned a basketful of numbers into a meaningful table or report may find themselves merely loading the data onto a VDT at a computer-paced speed and in a computer-determined order, while others turn that data into their final products.

VDTs, as they are being used in the typical office, are instruments of standardization, mechanization, and routinization, three reasons why they have been singled out by clerical workers' groups as a major threat to the respect and well-being of their constituencies. In *Race Against Time: Automation of the Office*, a concise analysis prepared by Working Women of the impact of automation on clericals, the authors write that "the first step towards the 'office of the future' is to apply the principles of factory production to office work."[11]

The office/factory analogy is right on target. More than 600 unique clerical and administrative tasks have been identified in offices, according to a study conducted by the Xerox Corporation.[12] More than 90 percent of those tasks are visual, and probably an equal proportion involve information processing, whether the "information" is in the form of words, numbers, or dollars. Xerox, along with a few hundred other companies concerned with the efficient workings of offices, is acutely aware of how computer technology has the potential to make virtually all of those 600 "tasks" operate more cost-efficiently. Such efficiency is achieved through isolating each task, breaking it down into its purpose, structure, and interaction (or lack of interaction) with other tasks. In the process, management efficiency experts hope to make the "whole" work better by improving each one of its parts.

Will it work? As we are beginning to learn, office automation may do more harm than good. One item not included in the sales pitches of computer manufacturers, automation consultants, or management consultants is the idea of "job content." It's a relatively simple notion: If a job seems impersonal and unstimulating, productivity and efficiency will be decreased no matter how much "productivity-improving" technology is introduced.

However simple it may be, this notion has eluded the bulk of business executives and office managers. "The people who make the systems changes in offices are systems-oriented people who have had little if any training in behavior," says John J. Connell, executive director of the Office Technology Research Group, a consortium of American, Canadian, and British executives who are studying the problems and promises of automation. "The behaviorists tend to be in the personnel department. There's a real need for education and communication between those two disciplines, but it's not happening. With all of the glamour and sex appeal of today's technology, executives often lose sight of the fact that we're not trying to automate the office — we're trying to improve productivity. The machines are, hopefully, tools to help in that task. But it's awfully easy to get so wrapped up in the machines that you forget the end purpose."

Indeed, office automation need not be a threat to clerical workers. It need not make work less interesting or more stressful. Computerized work actually can be extremely satisfying. For example, NIOSH, in its California study, found that professionals using VDTs complained of fewer ailments and professed considerably more job satisfaction. The reason, according to the researchers, was that "professionals using VDTs held jobs that allowed for flexibility, control over job tasks, utilization of their education, and a great deal of satisfaction and pride in their endproduct." In contrast, for the clerical VDT operators, "the VDT was part of a new technology that took more and more meaning out of the work."[13]

The NIOSH researchers concluded that the "working conditions that led to the stress problems reported by the clerical VDT operators are not entirely related to the VDT use, but are also related to the entire work system that goes along with using VDTs. In the case of the clerical VDT operators, the computer system technology under which they worked was designed without regard to the 'human' factor in the system."

"In essence," the report continued, "the design reflected the VDT and computer capabilities and performance functions which were then imposed on the operator. This is a serious concern since the persons who design systems such as these, and thereby the work activities of VDT operators, are typically computer scientists and systems analysts who have no concept of the human element in such a work process. This leads to dehumanization of the work activity that is similar to that produced by the introduction of assembly lines in manufacturing industries. In fact, such offices become 'paper factories' with clerical assembly lines....This leads to jobs that produce boredom and job dissatisfaction. As such, the machinery becomes a source of misery rather than a helpful tool...."

Such misery is evident in a Bell Telephone repair service office in Washington, D.C, as reported in *In These Times.* Workers at VDTs respond to telephone equipment repair requests, contacting repair crews via computer. Before the procedure was computerized, a worker's morning break came about two hours after the beginning of the shift; on the computerized printouts that list breaks and lunch times, some workers' morning breaks come within 15 minutes of arrival. Workers cannot go to the restroom without finding someone to take their place. "If you close your terminal," said one service representative, "right away the computer starts clacking away and starts ringing a bell." At the end of the day, a computer printout informs each supervisor of how many calls each clerk has taken and how often and for how long a terminal was abandoned.[14]

Such dehumanization is exacerbated by a major underlying concern of most office workers; the fear of "being replaced by a computer" has plagued workers — including many managers — almost since Day One of office computerization. The fear is not an irrational one. It's certainly no secret that word-processing equipment is aimed at eliminating as many workers as possible whose jobs are not based on "thinking." Today's word processors — which are still in their infancy stage, according to most industry experts — are capable of checking and correcting spelling, for example, and voice-activated systems are on the drawing boards of many leading-edge computer manufacturers.

Women will fare the worst in the era of computerization. According to Adam Osborne, in his book, *Running Wild: The Next Industrial Revolution,* more than 50 percent of today's jobs will be eliminated by the computer revolution during the next quarter century. Osborne says that computers will have their greatest impact in the same areas where women have made their greatest impact, and that five of every eight women workers are in an occupation that Osborne says will lose from 20 to 90 percent of existing jobs.[15] But it may be a lot sooner than 25 years before such trends become evident. According to a 1979 report on the office products industry prepared for the National Office Productions Association by SRI International, large organizations already are centralizing control over filing, word-processing, and data-handling operations.[16]

According to some projections, life may not be all that satisfying even for those who remain in the computerized offices of the future. Decreased job involvement, which is already concomitant with office technology, leads to increased anxiety about job roles, job advancement, and other key components of job satisfaction.

Adding to that anxiety is the relatively "lonely" atmosphere of the computerized office. Technology consultants promote computerization as something that decreases social interaction among clerical workers, supposedly a major roadblock to productivity and efficiency. With each employee at a computerized workstation, workers needn't commiserate as often at each other's desks, and there will be increasingly fewer reasons to travel to the "Xerox room" or to deliver memos or pick up mail by hand. The SRI report states that "there should be, in the early 1980s, the potential for more people to stay at their desk [sic] and yet utilize the same central office printing facility."

The SRI report notes that, in contrast to Japanese industry, which has developed corporate social institutions to promote worker interaction with other workers, "alienation of the [American] office worker is expected to be a growing problem." The report concludes that the office of the future "may quite possibly become a more impersonal place in which to work — it certainly will be quieter, more secure, and less expensively lighted, and this suggests a potentially far more lonely existence for the individual office worker."

The report adds an ominous warning: "We expect to see the office environment beset by a continual set of skirmishes between forces encouraging specialization and exchange, and forces encouraging the individual worker to do more of the task himself....If our analysis of the large office environment in the 1980s is correct, where the office environment is increasingly made up of a series of individual and very privately operated workstations, then there are considerable implications to management with regard to individual motivation, conveyance of team spirit, and

assistance in the individual worker's goal attainment."
The report might have added that such "considerable implications" to office managers often translate into considerable stress for office workers.

SOLVING VDT PROBLEMS

As the problems related to video display terminals begin to emerge and become more fully studied and defined, some solutions are emerging too. Unfortunately, the answers are coming considerably more slowly than the problems, and in many cases, they may be too late to get to the roots of the real problems involving VDTs.

Since little action has been taken by VDT manufacturers or by companies using the technology, most changes have come about due to a growing number of labor unions that have made VDTs a key health and safety issue. National union organizations with large VDT user populations — such as the Communication Workers of America, the Newspaper Guild, and the Office and Professional Employees International Union — have conducted seminars and educational campaigns, and have included VDT work requirements in bargaining contracts.

One key issue has been rest periods for VDT users — a practice that virtually every researcher has agreed can mitigate many of the hazards of VDT work. While no one knows exactly how long and how frequently breaks are needed to prevent VDT-related health problems, a number of researchers have offered specific suggestions that are likely to reduce some of the major complaints.

At a 1979 hearing before the California Industrial Welfare Commission, Andrea Hricko, then health coordinator of the Labor Occupational Health Program, outlined some examples:[17]

- Fatigue has been eliminated in radar operators who work for 140 minutes on screens, followed by a twenty-minute break.
- An Austrian trade union, on the basis of work performed at the University of Vienna, asked that workers doing "intensive work at machines be interrupted for fifteen minutes after maximally two hours; and that in

work involving continuous data screening equipment, a switch to a different activity should take place after one hour and continue for one hour."

● In Sweden, in some computerized offices, the operators have had so much muscle strain and eyestrain and felt so bored that they have refused to do certain terminal jobs for longer than two hours in the morning and two hours in the afternoon, and they have demanded and obtained job rotation.

● In Germany, agreements have been reached between banks and bank tellers for the following breaks: 10 minutes after 80 minutes of "feeding" the computer, and 10 minutes after 50 minutes of reading from the screen.

NIOSH, in the list of recommendations it issued following the California studies, recommended rest breaks "of at least fifteen minutes every two hours for VDT operators under moderate visual demands and fifteen minutes every hour for operators under high visual demands, high workload and...repetitive work tasks."

Some recommendations are even more conservative. For example, the British Association of Scientific, Technical and Managerial Staffs (ASTMS), in a formal "policy document," *Guide to Health Hazards of Visual Display Units*, recommended that during continuous VDT operation, "periods of work should not exceed two hours without a *half-hour break* and the maximum work in any day should be no more than four hours."[18] [emphasis added]

Even the nature of the breaks seems important. In line with employees' oft-stated preference for procedural flexibility, "informal," self-styled rest periods — as opposed to the more formal and structured rest periods preferred by many employers — produce the most benefits. This notion was confirmed by Gunnarsson and Soderberg's study of VDT workers at the Swedish Telecommunications Administration. The researchers concluded that "visual strain was more frequently observed among operators whose work was highly structured, inflexible, and done under conditions of stress. Those whose work had scope for formal breaks and varying tasks displayed fewer symptoms of visual strain. Of two groups, both taking formal breaks, one also took informal breaks and reported a lower degree of visual strain than the first group."

Unions in the United States and other countries have bargained for other conditions aimed at alleviating VDT-related problems. For example, in 1980, the Women's Caucus of the University of California, Berkeley chapter of the California State Employees' Association requested that:[19]

- A training program be provided to educate VDT operators about the machines;
- Instead of a separate full-time word processing category, operations of VDTs be incorporated into the clerical/administrative work category;
- No person work at a VDT terminal for more than four hours a day, with 15-minute rest breaks every 45 minutes;
- The university contract with an independent agency to monitor the health of VDT operators, and maintain health records during their employment;
- Eye examinations be provided to operators every six months, and corrective glasses be provided when supported by the recommendation of an optometrist or opthalmologist;
- Health training programs be provided;
- Equipment be provided to allow machines and chairs to be adjusted for individual operators; and
- All word processing equipment purchased include detached and adjustable screens with anti-reflective treatment and adjustable contrast and brightness controls.

The key ingredient to most of these solutions is *flexibility.* Keyboards should be separate from other components, allowing operators to position them for maximum comfort. Screens should be adjustable, both in up-down, left-right positions and in screen brightness. Chairs should be adjustable, to provide optimal seating position; ideally, the VDT operator should be able to look down slightly to view the screen.

Lighting should be adjustable, or at least dimmer than that of non-VDT workers. It should be dim enough to provide sufficient contrast of the images on the screen, yet bright enough to allow reading of a manuscript or other printed material. The optimum lighting, then, is a balance of the two needs. The British Association of Professional Executive and Computer Staffs, in a list of recommenda-

The NIOSH Recommendations

1. VDT workstations and devices should be made as flexible as possible to allow for individual operator control of:
   a. Keyboard height.
   b. Screen height.
   c. Screen brightness and contrast.
   d. Leg room.
   e. Viewing distance (should be within 450mm to 700mm).
   f. Workstation illumination levels (if indirect lighting at the workstation is provided).
   g. Chair adjustments (of the seat height, backrest height, and armrests).

2. The VDT screen should be position so that the viewing angle is 10° to 20° below the horizontal plane at eye level.

3. Illumination levels should be within 500 to 600 lux, with individual workstation lighting provided for jobs requiring higher levels due to visual demands.

4. Screen glare should be controlled through the use of any one or all of the following means:
   a. Windows should be covered with drapes or blinds to limit direct sunlight.
   b. VDTs should be positioned properly with respect to overhead lighting and high luminance sources in the work area.
   c. Hoods should be installed over screens to shield from direct or reflected light.
   d. A glare shield should be installed on the screen.
   e. Recessed lighting and special fixture covers should be used.

5. There should be mandatory work-rest breaks of at least fifteen minutes every two hours for VDT operators under moderate visual demands and ten minutes every hour for operators under high visual demands.

6. Visual testing of VDT operators should include:
   a. An initial complete opthalmologic examination including refraction, acuity, and accommodation testing; tests for color vision function; and examination of the cornea and the lens for opacity and the retina for detachment.
   b. Annual refraction, acuity, and accommodation testing.

tions contained in *Automation and the Office Worker,* put it this way: The amount of light hitting the screen "should be approximately half the level of luminance in a normal office...."[20] Recommendations vary widely, from 100 to 200 lux (about 10 to 20 footcandles) with additional task lighting added, recommended by Datapro Research Corporation, an office systems consultant,[21] to 500 to 600 lux (about 50 to 60 footcandles) with additional workstation lighting, in the NIOSH recommendations. Most important is that the light that reaches the VDT screen be reflected light, from walls and other surfaces, as opposed to direct light. But the reflections must be carefully directed onto the keyboard and printed material, and not into the VDT operator's eyes.

Some of the visual problems can be reduced by attachments to VDTs that make up for design deficiencies. Screens should be protected from reflections, either by a hood or by a matte finish that does not destroy image quality; anti-glare panels designed to fit over VDT screens can be used to minimize eye-straining reflections and glare. But screens and hoods won't eliminate glare and other lighting problems, only reduce them.

It shouldn't have to be said at all, but employer-employee communication is a key element in solving VDT-related problems, or avoiding them in the first place. ASTMS, the British association, in its *Guide to Health Hazards of Visual Display Units,* recommended that:[22]

- There should be full discussions with management on the introduction of the new technology. Major areas of job security, working hours, etc., should be agreed upon before detailed discussions are held on the design of the new system.
- Planning the introduction of the technology and new work patterns is essential, and full discussions should take place on the restructuring of jobs, limiting where possible the creation of a single category [VDT] operator.
- Agreement should be reached on the training program for all the workers involved in the reorganization. Training should include detailed information on how to adjust the working environment to suit the individual operator.

- There should be no agreement on work loads before a six-month trial period is completed by the operator. Agreements fixing rigid targets should be avoided. All agreements should attempt to maximize the control of the operator over the output.
- Joint management working groups should be set up to agree in detail on all points. It would make sense to set up a group to consider the environmental factors.

There are, of course, two kinds of solutions to VDT problems: low-technology (adjusting lighting, adding anti-glare screens, establishing rest periods, rotating job responsibilities, increasing employer-employee communications) and high-technology (redesigning the work structure, redesigning the physical environment, redesigning computer terminals). This distinction seems simple enough, but it is somehow forgotten in the arguments over the health effects of VDTs. Some of the most acute problems have rather workable solutions — ones that can satisfy a work force without turning an organization upside down.

Not that the high-tech problems should be ignored. They can't. Headaches, eyestrain, and sore backs result from a variety of interacting factors that must be considered as a whole. NIOSH, in its California study, concluded that "solutions for dealing with potential health problems posed by VDTs must encompass both job redesign and workplace redesign factors to deal with all the root causes of the problems. Additionally, the design of computerized office systems cannot be left solely to computer experts who are concerned mainly with the capabilities and needs of the machinery of the system, but must have significant impact from human factors experts who can take account of the needs of the 'people component' of the system."

NIOSH didn't say specifically, but the best "human factors experts" might just be VDT workers themselves.

CHAPTER FIVE

THE SLOW BURN

Of all of the pollutants known to twentieth-century humans, probably the most feared is something we've come to call "radiation." It is among the most insidious and deadly substances in the universe — and one of the least understood, particularly by the general public. The fears and the lack of knowledge are heightened by radiation's mysterious properties: it can't be touched, seen, smelled, or felt.

But it's there — everywhere. Radiation is as much a part of the universe as are the sun and the stars. In a variety of forms, it is contained in everything there is, including us. In some of its forms, it is harmless. In many of its forms, it is beneficial, even vital, to life on this planet. But in other forms, radiation poses a grave danger to human health.

With the introduction of office automation, some forms of radiation have invaded the office workplace. Video display terminals and other components of computer systems, as well as emerging microwave telecommunications systems and other technological wizardry, all are contributors. The amount of radiation they emit may be very small, but it is still of great concern, since we are just beginning to discover that low levels of radiation may be harmful.

This is an extremely touchy subject. Some of the world's largest corporations have a multi-billion-dollar stake in the office of the future, which includes computers, telecopiers, information storage and retrieval systems, satellite telecommunications, and other components of information-processing systems. Such systems already are in use, of course, although only in a small way, compared to the nature of the systems planned for the next few years.

That such technology could possibly be harmful is a subject that few manufacturers of such products are willing to discuss, let alone admit. Their equipment is safe, they'll quickly say, and challenge you to furnish proof to the contrary. Well, there is no concrete proof, but there is some disturbing evidence that should make computer users wary; some of that evidence has existed for as long as two decades. But the computer-industry giants remain largely unresponsive, at least publicly. They are helped along this path by a long line of government researchers and policymakers, who seem to have overlooked concerns for public health in favor of expediency, politics, or "national security."

Before we go into details, let's start with some basic principles and a brief history.

What exactly is "radiation"? The complete answer is extremely technical and not needed for this discussion. But here are a few basics. *Webster's New Twentieth Century Dictionary* (Second edition, unabridged) defines radiation as "the act or process of radiating; specifically, the process in which energy in the form of rays of light, heat, etc. is sent out from atoms and molecules as they undergo internal change."

Even that relatively straightforward definition is not that easy to understand, but it makes a good point: "radiation" is a variety of things. Visible light is radiation, as are heat and sound. Invisible ultraviolet light from the sun is another form of radiation. The electronic signals that we hear on the radio and see on television are two more forms of radiation. And, of course, the massive amounts of energy created during a nuclear bomb explosion and in the process of producing nuclear power are radiation.

Together, all of these forms of energy comprise the vast electromagnetic spectrum discussed in Chapter Three that includes x-rays, ultraviolet light, visible light, infra-

red light, microwaves, radio waves, and other components. Each segment of the spectrum represents energy
waves of specific lengths and frequencies of vibration.
(Frequency is expressed as the number of waves that pass
a given point in one second.) The shortest wavelengths are
0.0000000000003937 of an inch long, with frequencies of
billions of cycles per second; the longest waves measure
more than 3,000 miles, with frequencies of several thousand cycles per second. All are "radiation."

Soon after physicists understood the nature of electromagnetic waves, the spectrum was divided into two regions: "ionizing" and "nonionizing" radiation. The first
category includes gamma and x-rays, which have sufficient energy to dislodge electrons from atoms, creating
electrically charged atoms, called ions. Ionizing radiation,
because it damages the cells of living tissues, was found to
be capable of causing cancer and genetic mutations and,
therefore, to be very dangerous. Nonionizing radiation
was not considered to cause any harm.[1]

We now know how arbitrary that decision was. Over
the years, some researchers have found indications that
nonionizing radiation also has the potential for causing
harm, including possibly causing cataracts, genetic mutations, and cancer. More to the point: Given the right intensities and some other conducive conditions, it has been determined that *all* forms of electromagnetic radiation —
including radio frequencies, visible light, and other seemingly harmless segments — can be harmful to humans.

As surprising as these findings may seem, they have
been known for a long time. More than 50 years ago, for
example, Sir Stewart Duke-Elder, a British opthalmologist, demonstrated conclusively that rays originating anywhere throughout the electromagnetic spectrum were capable of causing cataracts. Moreover, he showed that the
cataract-forming effects of radiation, including sunlight,
were cumulative over many years. Finally, said Duke-
Elder, such radiation was the principal cause of most
types of cataracts.[2]

A cataract is a clouding of the lens within the eyeball,
which lies just behind the pupil. When healthy, the lens is
clear and pliable, and helps to focus the eye so that objects

can be seen sharply. Under certain conditions, the lens can harden and become cloudy, forming cataracts; the result is a blurring or clouding of vision, often accompanied by seeing multiple images or experiencing glare. Cataracts occur frequently in older people: of the approximately 325,000 people hospitalized for cataracts each year in the United States, 70 percent are over age 65. (More than 60 percent are women, a statistic that has never fully been understood.)[3]

Normal "aging" is the cause of the most common form of cataract, which occurs gradually, generally without any inflammation or pain. The process also occurs from minute exposures to radiation, which gradually heat the eyeball. The lens, when heated, becomes irreversibly opaque, much the same way an egg white does when it is cooked. A person need not even feel the radiation's heat for this to take place.

The phenomenon of microwave-induced cataracts has been known since the early 1950s, and the history of our understanding of the hazards of microwaves — and the subsequent cover-up that kept such information from the public for many years — is thoroughly and convincingly laid out in *The Zapping of America — Microwaves, Their Deadly Risk, and the Cover-up,* by Paul Brodeur, a staff writer for *New Yorker* magazine. Brodeur's book, published in 1977, is a shocking exposé. The book weaves the tale of the first suspected hazards of microwaves, which were used originally for radar and communications by the American military. The cover-up began as early as 1951, when a microwave technician employed under a government contract in New Mexico suffered severe cataracts, which were diagnosed by the attending physician as related to microwave radiation. Much of the cover-up was done in the name of "national security," since microwaves were an important component of our mobilization against the Russians during the 1950s Cold War. Early warnings about the hazards of microwaves by physicians and researchers were all but ignored by military and industrial policymakers, with the result that the American health standard for microwave radiation exposure was set *one thousand times* higher than that of the Soviet Union.

The Russians have been well aware of the hazards of radiation for many years. They ably demonstrated this by beaming microwaves into the American embassy in Moscow in the early 1960s, which resulted in embassy employees suffering nausea, bleeding of the eyes, and suspected chromosome damage; the history of the Russian microwave warfare is described in Brodeur's book. The U.S. Central Intelligence Agency, when it first learned of the Russian microwave assault, as well as of the substantial research done by the Russians on the effects of microwaves on human behavior, began intensive research of its own on the subject in 1962. The investigation was dubbed "Project Pandora," and the information about it was kept secret from everyone — including workers at the Moscow embassy.[4]

Among the people consulted during Project Pandora was Dr. Milton M. Zaret, an opthalmologist from Scarsdale, New York. Zaret had been investigating the effects of microwaves since 1959, when he began a study on the subject for the Defense Department. During the early 1960s, Zaret's studies of hundreds of microwave workers enabled him to arrive at some startling conclusions about the ability of microwave radiation to cause cataracts. In 1964, after he announced the results of a study linking microwaves and cataracts, the Air Force terminated his research. One Army opthalmologist told Zaret that "there was no such thing as a microwave cataract."[5]

In 1966, the American standard for occupational microwave exposure was set at ten milliwatts per square centimeter. (The power, or intensity, of microwaves and other electromagnetic radiation is customarily expressed as the amount of energy that flows each second through a square measure of space.) Zaret and others pointed to studies they had done showing that radiation levels as low as one milliwatt per square centimeter had produced cataracts. And the Soviets, who had conducted extensive research on the subject, set their exposure standard at one one-hundredth of a milliwatt, or one microwatt — one thousand times lower than the American standard. Some years later, the Chinese set their standard at 50 microwatts per square centimeter — 50 times higher than the

Soviet standard, but still 200 times more strict than the
American standard. Zaret maintains that all such standards are arbitrary, and that no level of radiation has yet
been proved safe. Zaret's detractors, including researchers
at NIOSH, maintain that the standards are adequate.

But Zaret's concern has been shared by others, including the authors of a 1971 White House report cited by Brodeur:[6]

> The electromagnetic radiations emanating from radar,
> television, communications systems, microwave ovens,
> industrial heat-treatment systems, medical diathermy
> units, and many other sources permeate the modern en-
> vironment, both civilian and military....This type of
> man-made radiation exposure has no counterpart in
> man's evolutionary background; it was relatively negli-
> gible prior to World War II....Power levels in and
> around American cities, airports, military installations,
> and tracking centers, ships and pleasure craft, indus-
> try and homes may already be biologically
> significant....The consequences of undervaluing or mis-
> judging the biological effects of long-term, low-level ex-
> posure could become a critical problem, especially if ge-
> netic effects are involved.

In early 1981, in the face of mounting evidence linking low-levels of microwave exposure with various ills, the
American National Standards Institute voted to adopt a
new microwave exposure limit of one milliwatt per square
centimeter, one-tenth the previous American standard.
However, many scientists feel that even the new standard
will, in turn, be replaced with one still more restrictive.[7]

What does all of this have to do with office workers?
Perhaps a great deal. On the basis of his work as one of
the foremost experts on the health effects of microwaves,
Dr. Zaret was called in to consult on a most interesting
case in 1977. Two copy editors at the *New York Times,*
aged 29 and 34, had acquired cataracts after about six
months of working on the newspaper's new video display
terminal system.

The two young men had been independently referred
to Zaret by their personal physicians. Zaret concluded that
both were suffering from cataracts "related to radiant en-

ergy injury of the intraocular lens" — in other words, both cases met Zaret's criteria for microwave-based cataracts. The Newspaper Guild hired Zaret as a consultant in the grievance proceedings of the two *Times* employees.

Meanwhile, the federal government also was called in on the case. The Center for Disease Control and NIOSH conducted an investigation of the *Times* facility. The results of those tests, which found levels of microwaves below the then-existing ten-milliwatt standard, were submitted to an arbitrator, who concluded that the *Times'* VDTs could not have caused the cataracts.

What, then, did cause the cataracts? The reports on the *Times* situation were confusing and contradictory. Arbitrator Maurice C. Benewitz concluded, based on the NIOSH evidence, that the cataracts also were compatible with those seen congenitally — existing at birth — or those associated with other causes. On the other hand, the NIOSH study did find levels of radiation that — while under the ten-milliwatt standard — were capable, according to Zaret and others, of producing cataracts. Moreover, the NIOSH investigation found that there had been hundreds of reports of malfunctions of the *Times'* VDT system, despite the *Times* management's contention that the machines were reliable. In the midst of such controversy, the actual cause was never determined. In March 1977, Zaret concluded in a letter to the Newspaper Guild, "The best that can be said about the NIOSH report is that it demonstrates serious faults of both commission and omission."

One big problem, says Zaret, was that what should have been a joint investigation between the Guild and the *Times* to determine the source of problems that were of concern to both, turned into a dogfight, with no one the winner. "When we discovered that there had been a large number of malfunctions in the *Times'* VDTs, there were immediate denials," says Zaret. "First from the manufacturer, then from the *Times* management. Everybody was assured that the equipment couldn't possibly under any circumstances emit radiation. Then it became very adversarial. Under adversarial conditions, you can't do a joint study."

In some cases, according to Zaret, the VDTs alone

weren't to blame, but had only contributed to the cataracts. An example was a 53-year-old female office worker Zaret examined who had been working with VDTs for four years. When referred to Zaret by her physician, she had been diagnosed as having a cataract in her right eye; two opthalmologists had ruled out all known causes of cataracts except radiation exposure. But Zaret, upon examination of the woman, found evidence that she had been exposed to radiation many years earlier, prior to her work with VDTs. After obtaining all of her medical records, he discovered that she had been given x-ray therapy on her face for acne, once an accepted form of therapy. Zaret concluded that the acne treatment had sensitized the lens of her eye and that the cataract was due "to the additive effect of the two different types of radiation" — the x-ray plus the VDT.

There have been other reports of radiation illnesses related to VDTs. Terminals at *Newsday* on Long Island were found to emit fifteen milliwatts of radiation, five milliwatts above the old safety standard and 1500 times the more conservative Soviet standard. The paper solved the problem by installing metal shields on the VDT units. *Computerworld,* in reporting the incident, noted that "no employees appear to have suffered any resulting health problems" — at least not in the first few days after the discovery. Perhaps a more accurate statement was made by a spokesman for Teleram, the manufacturer of the *Newsday* VDTs, who said that there was no "*immediate* danger to the health of employees."[8] [emphasis added]

In 1980, after two cataract cases developed among VDT users at the *Baltimore Sun,* the Newspaper Guild asked NIOSH to conduct an opthalmological study of the newspaper's 400 other VDT users. But the *Sun's* publisher was "anything but a model of cooperation," as Newspaper Guild president Charles A. Perlik Jr. told an investigative unit of the House Committee on Science and Technology, in hearings held in May 1981:

> After agreeing only with reluctance to go along with the NIOSH study (which NIOSH was in a position to enforce by court action), [the publisher] threw one roadblock after another in NIOSH's path. It declined for sev-

eral months to turn over the employee data NIOSH needed. It refused to let NIOSH into the plant to obtain employees' signatures on consent forms for the eye examinations, and when NIOSH set up a special van outside the plant for that purpose, it forbade employees to visit it during working hours. Only after NIOSH moved for a court order to gain access to the plant did the company agree to let the agency in...

Concern over VDT radiation also occurred in 1980 at the *Toronto Star,* after four employees of the newspaper's classified sales department gave birth to defective children during a three-month period. All four had worked on VDTs during the early months of their pregnancies, the most susceptible period for fetal deformation.

As in the *New York Times* case, there were immediate denials about the possibility of radiation at the *Star.* A spokesman for IBM, the manufacturer of the *Star's* VDTs, dismissed the connection between radiation and his company's product, saying that he considered the birth defects to be "totally new and without scientific predictability." The *Toronto Globe and Mail* quoted a NIOSH spokesman as saying that VDTs are "incapable of presenting high exposure that could cause fetal death or damage." Zaret and others contend that the levels need not necessarily be high to cause harmful effects.

Zaret, in a 1980 speech in France, summed up the situation like this:[9]

As if the [VDT] problem were not bad enough, its resolution is being hampered further by many different but not unrelated attempts for a quick fix. As gross equipment defects are found by crude testing, manufacturers, who previously denied there could be any problem, now pronounce these have been corrected by newly installed shielding (which didn't exist in the original model). NIOSH keeps citing its arbitrary, contrived standards for human exposure to nonionizing radiation as being safe while there is no ratiocinate reason to believe this to be true but, moreover, human pathology to affirm the opposite view. Labor and management, although it is in neither's long-term interest to do so, join each other in reassuring the workers with the palliative that there is little cause for concern. And, epidemiologists are attempting to ascertain how to keep score of the aftermath. Meanwhile, tragically, nothing meaningful is being accomplished regarding prevention."

To make matters worse, the results of the NIOSH investigation at the *New York Times* have been cited often as *the* authoritative view on VDTs and radiation. Another federal agency, the Food and Drug Administration's Bureau of Radiological Health, added to the misinformation in an article in the April 1981 issue of *FDA Consumer*. The article, entitled "VDTs Pass Medical Tests," tells of the bureau's testing of 125 VDTs for leakage of x-rays and other radiation. After noting that "problems were discovered in testing for x-ray leakage," the FDA concluded, "The consensus of the studies is that VDTs emit little or no harmful radiation under normal operating conditions." The agency also reported finding "insignificant" amounts of microwave and radio frequency radiation.[10] But John C. Villforth, director of the Bureau of Radiological Health, admitted in testimony before Congress in May 1981 that this conclusion was based only upon theoretical computer models; his agency had not actually performed any radiation tests. Dr. Zaret, who also testified at the hearing, called FDA's research methods "idiotic."

NEW FINDINGS

But what of the original concerns? Are microwaves produced by VDTs and other computer components harmful? If so, are there any safe levels? The answers to such questions remain largely unanswered, although researchers are gradually piecing together the evidence. And despite the new, tougher microwave exposure standards, the debate over worker safety rages on.

The core of one dispute is whether biological effects can be caused by *nonthermal* properties of microwaves. An assumption traditionally held by most experts was that nonionizing radiation could only effect living tissue by heating the tissue. Now, a growing body of evidence suggests that doses of radiation far below those that cause measurable heating can affect the growth of tissue, bone, and other living cells, can change brain-wave patterns, and can alter the action of enzymes that control nerve functions. Other effects of nonionizing radiation, according to scientific literature, include "cataracts, heart disease, infant deaths, damage to the immune system, depression, loss of memory, altered behavior, and a host of neurological disorders."[12]

One set of theories gaining credence in the scientific community says that low-frequencies of radiation — the kind emitted by VDTs and other electronic office equipment — interfere with the functioning of the brain. The most prominent of these theories maintains that our central nervous systems are extremely sensitive to man-made electromagnetic radiation in the environment, which interferes with the electromagnetic brain waves that can be observed on an electroencephalograph — a device used for measuring the electrical activity of the brain.[13]

Beginning in 1972, researchers demonstrated that low levels of microwaves could affect brain function. Dr. Suzanne Bawin and Dr. Rochelle Medici of the University of California at Los Angeles demonstrated that microwaves at one milliwatt per square centimeter could affect the behavior of cats; a Russian researcher, using a slightly higher level, was able to produce profound behavioral changes in mice. Other Russian scientists have shown that low levels of nonionizing radiation can cause fatigue, loss of sex drive, and irritability.[14] Even more to the point was a Chinese study of 1,312 workers, which showed that a group of people exposed to less than 200 microwatts had double the rate of neurological complaints as did a control group, as well as twice the rate of abnormal cardiac waves in men, and nearly ten times the rate of abnormal heartbeat.[15]

Most American scientists remain skeptical, contending that such experiments were poorly controlled, unreliable, and difficult or impossible to reproduce. But some American researchers believe that "the wholesale discounting of the Soviet and East European work is incorrect," according to Eric J. Lerner, writing in _Spectrum,_ a publication of the Institute of Electrical and Electronics

Engineers. "They feel that it is wrong to say that *none* of the several hundred published articles on low-level effects is sufficiently rigorous to be taken into account in the setting of a safety standard."[16]

In 1980, another concern emerged, although it was veiled amid a series of rules set forth by the Federal Communications Commission. The FCC, which is mandated with the responsibility of governing the use of the public airwaves through which radio and TV broadcasts travel, handed down a set of regulations prohibiting the sale of computing devices that emit unacceptable levels of radio-frequency interference, or RFI. The FCC defined a "computing device" to include digital telephone equipment and most data-processing equipment found in offices.

The FCC was concerned about RFI, not because of health and safety, but because the commission had received increasing complaints that RFI from computers was interfering with radio and television reception in some people's homes. As explained by Terry G. Mahn in *Byte,* a computer-industry magazine:[17]

> Computers and other similar devices emit potentially harmful radio-frequency signals. Inside a computer, very rapid electrical signals and pulses are generated and used to regulate sequences of events and to carry out the control and logic functions of the computer. These rapid electrical pulses produce high-frequency emissions that "float" around inside the cabinet of the computer. Unless this energy is somehow contained or filtered, it is radiated into space to be picked up by radio or television receivers.

One reason cited by Mahn for the growing number of interference complaints was "the increased replacement of steel [computer] cabinets with plastic cabinets, which provide little or no RFI shielding."

The FCC's concern is primarily with computers in residential settings, where interference with radio and TV signals poses the biggest problem. But the significance of the rule for the nation's office workers should not be overlooked. The FCC has recognized the growing amount of radio frequencies emanating from virtually all components of the electronic office, including electric wires connecting computer terminals with central storage devices; security systems; computerized heating and cooling management systems; and telecommunications systems, including many of the growing number of private long-distance telephone systems.

In a manner similar to microwaves, radio-frequency (RF) radiation can have harmful effects on humans, although such effects are not within the Federal Communications Commission's sphere of interest. Like microwaves, RF radiation has been implicated as being able to produce cataracts, and may be a factor in other adverse health effects. But unlike the relatively conclusive evidence linking microwaves with adverse health effects, there is extremely little known about the amounts of RF that can be harmful, and whether low levels found in offices can cause ill effects over prolonged periods.

Additional study is clearly needed in light of the skyrocketing increase in RF use in office buildings. And use of RF-generating equipment will increase even more in coming years. Already, some buildings are being constructed with higher voltage electric wires that can accommodate increased use of computers; one example is the Ethernet Network created by the Xerox Corporation, which enables a business to plug computer terminals, printers, and storage devices into handy "information outlets" mounted on the wall, much like you now plug your TV into an AC electrical outlet." At Dow Jones & Company, publisher of the *Wall Street Journal*, experimental circuits are being used to relay news in digital (computerized) form over telephone lines and through electric wiring to computer terminals and teleprinters scattered about its New York City offices.

More than a dozen new satellite communications networks are either "on-line" or in the works, involving such corporate behemoths as IBM, AT&T, Western Union, RCA, Southern Pacific, MCI, GTE, and several other major American companies. Most such systems utilize both microwaves and radio frequencies in the transmission of voice- and data-communications throughout offices and across oceans. In many cases, the systems use "dish" antennas mounted on rooftops and in parking lots, although there are few rules governing leakage of radiation from such dishes and from other components of the systems. And no new regulations are planned.

New rules might not even be necessary, but that's just the point: No one really knows for certain what effects, if any, this vast new input of RF and microwave radiation might have on the people who use them — and the people who just happen to work in the area.

Concern over such information gaps is just beginning to build. With the lack of conclusive information that exists, there is little that most workers can do, other than to be aware of the possibilities. Calling in federal inspectors doesn't do much good, either. "Our position is that it doesn't do unions any good to call us in if we're just taking environmental measurements," says one OSHA official. "Because we'll just go in and take measurements and, sure enough, the levels will be way, way below any existing or proposed standards. However, if there's a scientific study that indicates an increased incidence of some problems, then we can take action." But that scientific study has yet to be made. The Newspaper Guild and Communications Workers of America — two unions with members who use VDTs extensively — are leading the cry for new and definitive studies on the effects of VDTs in offices; no union has yet expressed any concern over other potentially harmful aspects of the electronic office. Everyone concerned seems to realize that the answers will be slow in coming. One Newspaper Guild representative expressed the concerns of many when he said, "This whole thing may end up like Three Mile Island: We won't know the damage for another ten or twenty years."

CHAPTER SIX

STRESSED TO KILL

Until recently, occupational stress was simply not associated with office work. In the Louis Harris survey, in which a thousand office workers were asked a few dozen questions about their comfort and productivity, the pollsters never even raised the subject of stress. Traditionally, stressful jobs were thought to be held by assembly-line workers, stock traders, chief executive officers, fire fighters, and politicians — in other words, anyone who had a job that was high-pressured, involving long hours and fast-paced work. The secretary or receptionist was not considered to be in this category.

That myth has gone the way of the manual typewriter. Increasingly, we're finding that such seemingly mundane jobs as secretarial and clerical work can produce physical and psychological ailments that have come to be known as "stress-related" illnesses. And the more we're learning about stress at work, the more we're finding that secretarial and clerical jobs may be among the most stressful jobs around.

A lot of what's being discovered about office work and stress is an extension of studies done of blue-collar workers a half-century ago. For example, in a classic work published in 1932, *Workers Emotions in Shop and Home*, Rex Hersey described the broad range of "sources of crises" that created stress among blue-collar workers:[1]

...the work itself, including the nature of the job, the amount accomplished, plant conditions, treatment by the foremen, relations with one's fellow workers, etc; the physical condition of the worker, including a source which, for want of a better term, we may call "inside feeling"; outside causes, including relations with wife and children, influences of parents, success with girls, anticipation or memory of parties and other attempts at recreation, etc.; finances; and, finally, weather.

The comparison between stress in offices and in factories is appropriate. As office work becomes more mechanized, with computer technology creeping into most aspects of office work, an emerging office assembly line is producing many of the adverse psychological health effects of the blue-collar worker. "The office of the future is a recreation of the factory of the past," is a favorite slogan of office-workers' rights groups. The whirring, pounding, and drilling of the factory or coal mine may not exist in the office (although there is still noise-related stress in offices), but many of the same problems facing office workers replicate those of their blue-collar brethren.

Fifty years after Rex Hersey's book, the potential "sources of crises" he described exist for office workers, as well as for most factory workers, although as life has gotten more varied and complex, so have the stressors. As in Hersey's factory of the 1930s, job stress among modern office workers in the 1980s may be attributed to physical factors (noise, lights, video display terminals), the nature of the job (sexual harassment, boring work, machine-paced tasks, lack of job security), personal factors (family life; social life; relations with colleagues, bosses, and subordinates), societal factors ("keeping up with the Joneses") and — yes — the weather.

In April 1981, Working Women released the results of a survey of nearly 1,000 office workers in Boston and Cleveland, concluding that there is "a virtual epidemic of stress symptoms and stress-related disease among office workers." In the survey, 72.5 percent of the respondents reported "somewhat stressful" or "very stressful" working conditions; the sources of stress are summarized in the table on the following page.[2]

Perhaps it is a sign of the times, but "stress" has become a hot topic in the 1980s. Bookstore shelves and mag-

Sources of Stress in Office Jobs

Source	Rate
Lack of promotions or raises	51.7%
Low pay	49.0
Monotonous, repetitive work	40.0
No input into decision-making	35.1
Heavy workload/overtime	31.5
Supervision problems	30.6
Unclear job descriptions	30.2
Unsupportive boss	28.1
Inability/reluctance to express frustration or anger	22.8
Production quotas	22.4
Difficulty juggling home/family responsibilities	12.8
Inadequate breaks	12.6
Sexual harassment	5.6

Source: Answers by 915 respondents to survey conducted in Boston and Cleveland by Working Women Education Fund, Fall, 1980.

azine racks are brimming with tomes on managing stress, coping with stress, eliminating stress, and thriving with stress. Stress-education projects are being set up by a growing number of unions and occupational safety and health groups to identify stress problems and suggest remedies. Stress management consulting is a booming business — particularly in trend-setting California — with professional advisors teaching executives, supervisors, and workers how to minimize and even counteract the stresses of everyday work life. High-priced seminars for managers and executives are held on a daily basis around the country ("How to thrive on the pressures of life in the corporate world," is the title of one recent program — $145 for a one-day seminar plus workbook). Clearly, we have become the best-stressed society in human history.

As commonly as the term "stress" is used, however, it is frequently misused, or at least misunderstood. "Stress" is generally thought to refer to psychological pressure, to worrying, to bad times. This isn't incorrect, but it isn't entirely true either.

Granted, "stress" is not an easy concept to explain or to understand. Dr. Hans Selye, author of *The Stress of Life* and numerous other books on the subject, is probably the most respected authority on stress. Selye begins his definition of "stress" by explaining what it is *not*. For example, says Selye:[3]

- Stress is *not* simply nervous tension.
- Stress is *not* an emergency discharge of adrenaline.
- Stress is *not* anything that causes an alarm reaction.
- Stress is *not* necessarily something bad.
- Stress *cannot* and *should not* be avoided.

Selye defines stress as "the nonspecific response of the body to any demand made upon it." Put another way, stress is the body's way of reacting to normal and abnormal occurrences in order to keep the body functioning smoothly and to protect it from harm.

Stress is a vital part of being alive. When we exercise, we stress our muscles and our heart. When our intestines digest last night's dinner, they are stressed. A cut or an infection or an allergy creates stress on certain parts of our system. Stress is the normal wear and tear of everyday life. But, as Selye points out, there is good stress and there is harmful stress; he refers to them as "eustress" and "distress." Even more confusing is that some "stressful" activities may not be harmful, and some good things may cause harmful stress: You can get ulcers from being too happy. Selye's example:[4]

> The mother who is suddenly told that her only son died in battle suffers a terrible mental shock; if years later it turns out that the news was false and the son unexpectedly walks into her room alive and well, she experiences extreme joy. The specific results of the two events, sorrow and joy, are completely different, in fact, opposite to each other, yet their stressor effect — the nonspecific demand to readjust herself to an entirely new situation — may be the same.

Stress is not totally dependent on a psychological state; it doesn't matter whether or not you *think* you are under pressure or are bothered about something to become stressed. Stress is a physical response to one or more stressors, whether you are aware of them or not. Your body, ever vigilant, watches out for stressors.

Regardless of the source of the stress, there are some common physical reactions that often occur during stressful situations: your breathing and heartbeat increase; there is an increase in the secretion of stomach acid and of hormones that affect metabolism. In more extreme cases, there is an emergency release of adrenaline, as well as a rise in cholesterol and sugar levels in your blood. The increased energy from the higher blood sugar goes to your muscles, often creating tension. The reaction is most often felt in your stomach (the site of most "gut" reactions), which becomes inactive during this process. You may get queasy, "butterflies," nauseous, a stomachache, or simply lose your appetite.

In most normal situations, the body returns to a balanced state after the stressful situation has subsided. But over a prolonged period, or after frequent occurrences, these protective mechanisms of the body can begin to cause harm. One of the better known effects is the higher level of cholesterol in the blood of a stressed individual — a major contributor to coronary heart disease. Other illnesses commonly associated with stress are hypertension, ulcers, and nervous disorders.

Numerous other ailments have been associated with stress, from bursitis to balding. For example, "Stress can have a profound effect on dental health," according to Dr. William Howard, a professor at the school of dentistry at the University of Oregon. Howard says that the chemical reactions resulting from stress accelerate the development of periodontal disease, such as infection and erosion of the gums and bones that support the teeth. In addition, gnashing and grinding of the teeth — known as "bruxism" — which is a common trait of stressed individuals, can result in the wearing down, cracking, and even breaking of teeth. It can also cause headaches, backaches, and severe facial pain.[5]

Another recent finding is that stress may be addictive. According to Waino Soujanen, a professor at Georgia State University in Atlanta, and Donald Hudson, a professor at the University of Miami in Florida, "Without realizing it, many of us...are just as dependent on the 'high' we get from earning our daily bread as the 'speed freak' is on his pills." The two researchers believe that some people have a predisposition to become hooked on the adrenaline hormone produced during stressful situations, and that the adrenaline "fix" closely resembles that of amphetamines, or "speed." And like the drug addict, the "stress freak" needs bigger and bigger doses of the hormone. As a result, some people try "to build fires in order to put them out, or manufacture crises [they] can stand up under," according to Soujanen and Hudson.[6]

MEN, WOMEN, AND STRESS

How stressful is office work? Part of the answer has to do with your gender and your family life, according to the results of a study released in 1980 by Drs. Suzanne G. Haynes and Manning Feinleib of the National Heart, Lung, and Blood Institute, part of the National Institutes of Health. The study was a part of the "Framingham Heart Study," a project that has followed the fates of more than 1,300 men and women for over twenty years, keeping track of their heart attacks, chest pains, and other symptoms of coronary heart disease (CHD); this segment of the larger study involved an eight-year period. The subjects included 580 men, 350 housewives, and 387 working women, all of whom were free of coronary heart disease at the start of the study. More than one-third of the working women studied had been employed in clerical and other similar office occupations during their working years — for example, as secretaries, stenographers, bookkeepers, bank clerks and cashiers, and sales personnel; this percentage parallels the make-up of the overall national work force.[7]

Haynes and Feinleib found that women clerical workers developed CHD at almost twice the rate as other white- or blue-collar female workers or housewives.

Among men, the pattern was entirely different, with male clerical workers experiencing about one-fourth the rate of CHD as other male white-collar workers, and less than half that of male blue-collar workers.

Among women clericals, those who married were at greater risk of developing coronary heart disease, and the incidence rose as the number of children they had increased. Moreover, "single married clerical workers without children were at no greater risk of developing CHD than other workers," according to Haynes and Feinleib. "These findings suggest that the dual roles of employment and raising a family may produce excessive demands on working women."

There were other contributors to CHD among clericals. Haynes and Feinleib wrote, "Clerical workers who developed CHD were more likely to suppress hostility...to have a nonsupportive boss, to report fewer personal worries, and to experience fewer job changes over a previous ten-year period than clerical workers remaining free of CHD."

"Thus," they concluded, "remaining in a job with a nonsupportive boss while not discussing one's anger increased the risk of coronary heart disease among clerical working women. This risk was further increased with the size of the family."

The Framingham study was not the first to link office work with stress-related illnesses, particularly among women. As Haynes and Feinleib pointed out, "These findings are consistent with observations that women clerical workers may experience several forms of occupational stress, including a lack of autonomy and control over the work environment, underutilization of skills, and a lack of recognition of accomplishments."

Another study, conducted by NIOSH in 1977, looked at death certificates, hospital admissions, and mental-health center admissions of more than 22,000 Tennessee residents in 130 occupations in order to correlate jobs to stress-related illness. Among the twelve occupations singled out as displaying "very significant incident rates," secretaries were ranked second just behind laborers, and just ahead of inspectors, clinical laboratory technicians, and office managers. "One of the most interesting aspects of evaluating all of the high stress-related disease incidence occupations, which vary widely in their job requirements, is the similarity of certain stressors in these occupations," wrote the study's authors. "For instance, most all of these occupations require a fast workpace with little chance of relief from the pace. Many of these occupations require long working hours, repetitive and/or boring job tasks and produce an overall feeling of pressure, tension, and anxiety without outlets for these feelings."[8]

Of course, such job characteristics create stress in higher-level office jobs too, particularly among women. In 1980, Drs. Laraine T. Zappert and Harvey M. Weinstein of Stanford University reported on their study of recent business school graduates. The two researchers sent questionnaires to an equal number of male and female Masters of Business Administration (MBA) graduates from the 1977 and 1978 classes of "a large and prestigious graduate business school," in order to measure work stress and health status. Both the men and the women reported having a great deal of authority, responsibility, and autonomy in their jobs, and all said they had respect from supervisors and co-workers. But when asked "How stressful is your job?", women more often reported feeling bound by inflexible time schedules, felt unable to control the work flow to their satisfaction, and more often found their work to be boring.[9]

Zappert and Weinstein also found big differences in physical and psychological ailments between the men and women in their study. "Physically, women reported being more often bothered by stomach upsets and a variety of nonspecific ailments," they wrote. "Women also reported significantly more psychological distress focused on feelings of depression, nightmares, feeling overwhelmed, feeling on the verge of a nervous breakdown, and feeling that life was too much for them." They found that four times as many women as men "had seen mental health professionals in the past three years," and concluded that "both the work environment and conflicting demands between home and work may be contributing to these findings."

The link between stress at work and stress at home is

often overlooked. The two stresses have a synergistic effect — that is, they feed off of each other, making each situation even more stressful than it already is. Dr. Elliott Liebow of the Center for Work and Mental Health at the National Institute of Mental Health, explained it like this:[10]

> Job stress may be a very personal experience, but it is by no means a private one. It's crucial to realize that the stress experienced by the worker and his or her reaction to them — depression, anxiety, anger, boredom, shame — or respiratory, blood pressure, or stomach problems — that these things do not stay in the workplace. The worker takes them home, where they shape his or her relationship with his or her family and friends....These stresses are diffused throughout the community. After a while the worker, or members of his or her family, becomes a statistic, having to do with alcohol or drug abuse, physical illness, mental illness, family break-up, violence, or something else. And *then* the worker may even become one of those "troubled workers" who brings his [sic] problems with him into the workplace.

Of course, the economic realities of the day have made the employment game a buyer's market, with most companies preferring to get rid of "troublemakers" who offer suggestions to make office life less stressful, let alone more satisfying. For the majority of women office workers, "job satisfaction" is an elusive dream, overshadowed by economic concerns. Most women work out of necessity: two-thirds of all married female clerical workers have husbands who earned $10,000 or less in 1979.[11]

Even among the more financially fortunate clericals and secretaries, job satisfaction is still less than bountiful — again, particularly among women. A survey by the Department of Labor in 1971 found that women are nearly twice as likely to be dissatisfied with their jobs as men, due mostly to matters of salaries and promotional opportunities.[12]

MACHINE-PACED WORK

As noted in Chapter Four, office automation equipment may be causing more problems than it solves, at least as far as worker health and safety are concerned. In addition to the wide range of physiological problems that video display terminals create, or are suspected of creating, there are many psychological stressors associated with VDTs. Among the more serious ones are the monotony, boredom, and inflexibility created by the work pace dictated by many video display terminal systems.

Consider the following scenarios, found with increasing frequency in American offices:

- At a large Illinois insurance company, "claim processors" take phone calls from customers. The phone calls are automatically routed to them via a computerized telephone switching device. As soon as the claim is processed, another one appears. Meanwhile, supervisors monitor the speed and accuracy of workers with their own computer terminals, which provide instant information on the number of calls handled and the length of each call.
- At a bank in Dallas, clerks spend eight hours a day processing loan applications on video display terminals. Each clerk is responsible for inserting and coding five to seven pieces of information. As soon as the information is completed, the form automatically disappears, and a new one comes up on the screen. Supervisors, meanwhile, can monitor the number of strokes per second for each clerk, and each clerk's daily record is maintained in individual employee files.
- Just outside of Boston, in a telephone company service center, "communications consultants" process customer orders on VDTs. Company policy dictates that each worker report for work, take breaks, and eat lunch according to an assigned schedule. At the designated times, the computer screens automatically notify workers that it is time to take a break; the computers report to supervisors exactly what time breaks begin and end, and other times that employees sign on or off the machines.
- At a magazine subscription service center in Colorado, employees work full-time on VDTs processing subscriptions and changing addresses. In 1980, when the computers were introduced, workers' hourly wages were ended, with each employee paid instead by the number of subscriptions processed per eight-hour shift.

As the above examples indicate, automation is taking control of employees' working lives in some offices, contributing to feelings of alienation and job dissatisfaction that already exist among lower-paid workers. As Barbara Pottgen, claims examiner for Blue Cross/Blue Shield in San Francisco put it: "There is no room for creativity in my job performance. Opportunities to talk with other people have been virtually eliminated....This has increased the amount of control that management has over my work routine."[13]

In their 1980 study of office worker health problems, Working Women concluded that machine pacing and work speed-ups are "very powerful factors in stress-related symptoms." As an example, they cite the testimony of "an eight-year employee of the data-entry department of a large Cleveland utility" who experienced a "speed-up" mandate by management:[14]

> We used to have to process a maximum of 4,000 checks a day. Now, 4,000 has become the minimum — that's one check every six seconds — and the average they require is between 5,000 and 6,000 — about four seconds per check. Now, they are treating us like machines, expecting that everyone can do exactly the same amount every day, no matter how hard or easy checks are to process. It's hard to keep your temper from flaring when you're so tense about meeting production quotas.

Such working conditions — combined with long working hours, monotony, lack of recognition and respect, and an unsupportive boss — become the building blocks of stress: as the problems add up, the probability of stress-related emotional or physical problems increases.

Dr. Michael Smith, a NIOSH psychologist who has studied the effects of VDTs on worker stress, confirms, "These jobs are repetitious and every little keystroke that an individual makes is recorded by the computer and a supervisor has only to look into a video tube to be able to key in on particular individuals and their performance. Partly as a result of this, VDT operators have the highest stress jobs that we've ever seen — and we've been in the stress business for ten years."

Which is not to say that video display terminals and

the other components of office automation need necessarily be banned. There's little question that such devices have the potential to make work easier for everyone — which, in turn, can have a positive effect on productivity and job satisfaction. Unfortunately, that's not often the case.

NO NOISE IS GOOD NOISE

As one legal secretary put it: "You can't hear yourself think. But you can hear everyone else."

Until recently, there had been very little concern about the effects of noise in offices. In fact, thanks to automation, the overall level of office noise has diminished in most offices — the clanging of typewriters, adding machines, and mimeograph machines has been replaced with the soft *whrrrr* of video display terminals, calculators, and photocopiers.

Despite the relative quiet, office workers do have some noise problems. The problems are different from those of the jackhammer operator, the factory worker, or the rock musician, who experience prolonged exposure to high noise levels that can damage ears enough to cause permanent hearing loss. That's not the problem in most modern offices, although it does exist in some.

What exactly is "noise"? The classic definition is "unwanted sound." That definition has little to do with extreme loudness — it's the *relative* level of sound that's important. Dropping a heavy book on a wooden floor would not be jarring in the middle of a crowded bookstore; in a quiet library it would probably be a major disruption. Similarly, an animated conversation might not be noticed in a restaurant; in the middle of an open office, it could cause virtually all productive work to cease.

In other words, the intensity of noise is not merely how loud it is, but how unwanted it is, and how unexpected it is.

The human ear is an ever-vigilant organ. Unlike the eye, which has an automatic control mechanism to regulate the amount of light entering it, the ear remains fully open all of the time. Even when sleeping, our ears remain

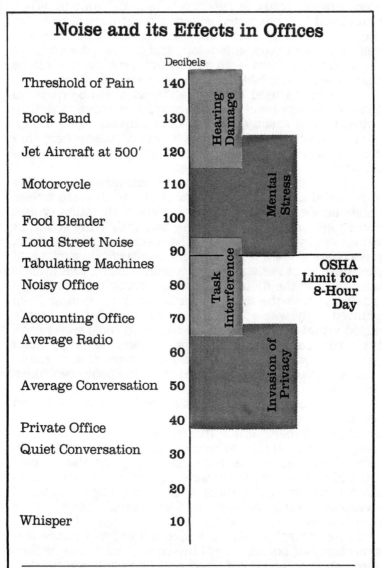

Noise and its Effects in Offices

Decibels

Threshold of Pain	140
Rock Band	130
Jet Aircraft at 500'	120
Motorcycle	110
Food Blender	100
Loud Street Noise	
Tabulating Machines	90
Noisy Office	80
Accounting Office	70
Average Radio	60
Average Conversation	50
Private Office	40
Quiet Conversation	30
	20
Whisper	10

Hearing Damage

Mental Stress

Task Interference

Invasion of Privacy

OSHA Limit for 8-Hour Day

Source: _Noise and Office Work_, by Susan T. Mackenzie (Cornell University, 1975), and other sources.

alert, always ready to respond to unusual sounds. When stimulated by unexpected sound, a physiological response occurs in the rest of the body: increased blood pressure, heartbeat, and muscle tension, and decreased activity of the digestive system — in other words, the basic reactions that have come to be known as symptoms of "stress."

We can get used to noise, although that doesn't mean that the stress reactions go away. There is conflicting opinion about exactly what effect continuous noise has on mental health; it is suspected by many researchers that continuous noise is less of a problem than sudden, irregular noises.

One study that looked into the minutiae of everyday secretarial life illustrated how these unexpected noises create stress. Two groups of workers — dictation typists and receptionist/copy typists — had their daily activities monitored by TV cameras for the researchers. In addition, physiological tests were given for cardiac frequency, blood pressure, skin resistance, skin temperature, and muscle tension. For the dictation typists, typing from dictation machines was the least-stressful activity; typing from printed copy was somewhat more stressful due to the added visual demands. For the reception room secretaries, typing in general was the least-stressful activity; much greater stress resulted from a startled reaction to noise, such as having the telephone ring or the door open unexpectedly.[15]

More recently, researchers at the University of Miami School of Medicine studied the effects of everyday noise on monkeys. Experimental animals were exposed continuously for nine months to recordings of the sounds an ordinary blue-collar worker encounters daily: an alarm clock, a flushing toilet, running water, gargling, shaving, a radio playing, twenty minutes of the *Today* show, sounds of a construction project, a televised football game, an air conditioner, and a few distant motorcycles. Compared with the control monkeys, which did not experience this symphony of sound, the "blue-collar" monkeys experienced an average rise of blood pressure of 27 percent during the study period. Moreover, the blood pressure remained high long after the noises stopped.[16]

The monkeys aren't human, of course, and their noise exposure wasn't that of offices, but the study did show that sustained elevated blood pressure can result from long periods of noise not loud enough to have any adverse effects on hearing. The fact that those intermittent noises produced stress long after the noises ended does not bode well for the many office workers who endure periodic noise throughout the day from people and machines.

Loud noises do exist in offices. In a room with five or more typewriters or copiers operating simultaneously, noise can exceed the levels recommended for work involving verbal communications.[17] Office tabulating machines have been measured at 80 decibels or more, and addressographs at 90 decibels. High-speed printers attached to computer terminals can make quite a racket, making intellectual work difficult for workers in the general vicinity. Offices located within industrial settings have noise problems too: at a General Electric facility in Ohio, workers in an office adjacent to the factory were distracted by machine noise coming through walls; the sound was measured at around 75 decibels.[18] The Occupational Safety and Health Administration has set limits of 90 decibels for an eight-hour day, although some scientists believe that lower levels can cause physiological problems as well. Such noise levels may tire out the inner ear, causing temporary reductions in hearing ability; after a period of relative quiet, the hearing ability is usually restored. With continuous noise exposure, the ear can suffer permanent hearing damage.

It's not as if producing quieter office products isn't technologically possible: According to one manufacturer of typewriters, the cost of adding sound-deadening materials to an electric typewriter was only around 60 cents.[19]

One major source of noise in offices is people talking. Sounds from conversations carry — across rooms, between walls, and through open doors. Usually, the level of the conversation isn't as distracting as being able to understand the words, which can be devastating to an individual who is trying to concentrate.

Persistent noise can be a big problem in the "open" or "landscaped" office, where partitions are used instead of walls to create individual "workstations." The typical partition stands about five to six feet high, and may or may not touch the floor all along its length. It may be covered with steel, carpet, plastic, or any of a dozen other materials. Few partitions absorb sound effectively.

One Wall Street law firm experienced a 54 percent turnover of employees, which was later attributed largely to problems with noise. Almost a hundred people, each with a telephone, were crammed into a single office. Speech communication and telephone conversations — the two principal activities in that workplace — were made extremely difficult. Time lost during the work day required the company to utilize a lot of worker overtime. The problem was significantly reduced by the installation of sound absorbent material on the ceiling and floor, and a rearrangement of workers according to communications patterns. Telephone bells were reduced to one bell per table, with lighted buttons identifying individual lines in use.[20]

Sounds travel through open offices in three different ways: directly through space dividers or partitions; by being reflected off the ceiling (particularly off of plastic panels covering fluorescent lighting fixtures) above one partition and into an adjacent office; or by diffraction — like light rays — hovering over, under, and around partitions and into other offices. The result: You hear conversations taking place next door and across the room; you can't tell whose telephone is ringing; you waste a lot of time being angry. Even executives in private offices are victims of noise distractions: A survey conducted for the Omega Watch Corporation found that 43 percent of major corporate chief executive officers considered normal office hours were a terrible time to get anything done. They preferred the hours before 9 AM and after 5 PM.

Some offices have minimized the effects of noise by using a "masking" sound. Most common is "white noise" — similar to the sounds of a fountain or of a television tuned to a nonbroadcasting station. But such systems are not always effective and some people are disturbed by the masking noise as well. Bitter battles have ensued in offices where employees take turns adjusting the master volume control of the masking sound. In a building recently constructed for the Department of Health and Human Services in Washington, D.C., a $100,000 masking system was shut off completely after only a few months due to worker complaints.

Another masking sound is Muzak. Everybody knows Muzak as the carefully controlled musical sounds that emanate from elevators, shopping centers, dentists' offices, on the telephone when placed on "hold" — and in offices.

The idea of using music to stimulate productivity and efficiency is not new; it began nearly a century ago in factories when employers hired live bands, orchestras, and choruses to inspire workers. (Actually, live music in factories has had something of a revival. In 1980, the John Deere Co., a farm equipment manufacturer, hired a concert pianist to present recitals so that factory assembly-line workers could enjoy music during lunch and coffee breaks.) With the advent of public address systems, music in factories became commonplace.

Music in offices is nothing short of a science. Muzak Corporation's "board of scientific advisors" creates carefully programmed music that is, as they put it, "heard, but not listened to." The company creates all of its own music in its recording studios. By controlling orchestra size and the music's rhythm and tempo, Muzak claims to influence body, mind, and emotion on both conscious and unconscious levels. It works like this: Programs are planned in fifteen-minute segments. Each segment is divided into three, five-minute subsegments that increase in tempo and rhythm during each quarter-hour. Fifteen-minute segments are altered with periods of silence. As one New York office worker described it: "In the morning, we listen to a soft pseudo-rock concert, but after three o'clock, the music gets rockier and louder."[21] All this goes on 24 hours a day, 365 days a year. Muzak programs are never repeated; each day, used Muzak programs are shipped to other cities, or transmitted over airwaves and telephone lines.

Muzak's marketing claims are just slightly short of Orwellian. Consider: "We can change your heartbeat...affect your metabolism and respiration...increase or decrease energy and alertness...make you feel relaxed or excited." In offices, Muzak claims that it "enhances employee morale ... actually makes their work more interesting...increases employee alertness...reduces boredom caused by monotonous routine...creates a sense of management caring."

In fact, there is no clear-cut evidence that piped in music can accomplish these things. Muzak boasts productivity-improvement studies, but they are inconclusive. An independent study, performed at an Australian university in 1969, concluded that "background music had no significant sustained effect on either work rates or error rates," although the majority of the employees preferred the background music over no music.[22] But there also are those vehemently opposed to the piped-in music: At the midtown Manhattan offices of snooty *New Yorker* magazine, for example, workers threatened to walk out if the building owner refused to turn off the Muzak in the elevator.[23]

CROWDING: A SPACE ODYSSEY

In many big cities, office space is a dear commodity. In New York City, for example, leased office space in new buildings went for up to $70 per square foot in mid-1981, and rents were high in other cities and suburbs as well. A study released in 1980 found that, despite an apparent boom in office building construction, the actual supply of office space is shrinking.[24] For management, the challenge of the 1980s is to do more business in less space. For office workers, "doing more in less space" means less elbow room per worker, less total work space, fewer amenities — such as lunchrooms or lounges — and more crowding.

According to one study, increased density isn't necessarily bad. A study of 100 "office workers in the headquarters of a major corporation" found increased worker satisfaction when work spaces were moved closer together; the workers cited "increased feedback," which "gave the employees increased chances to 'check signals,' share expectations, and to both give and receive informal feedback on task performance." Increased social density also produced an increase in workers' abilities to develop friendships among fellow workers.[25] Robert Propst, the father of the modern open office, agrees: "One of the great assets of a more frankly interactive and open office expression is the improved social structure it offers," he wrote in _The Office — A Facility Based on Change._ He notes that "we all have a fear of being lost from view, forgotten, bypassed, and left out" — fears that are presumably eased in the open office.[26]

But not everyone agrees with that analysis. Robert Sommer, in his book _Tight Spaces — Hard Architecture and How to Humanize It,_ writes that, "Crowding by itself does not increase communication or social contact. Indeed, it may strengthen a social order that discourages communication in order to prevent overstimulation from too many people in too little space."[27] A number of studies have correlated crowding with high blood pressure in humans.[28] When animals are crowded, death rates increase, reproductive cycles are disrupted, sexual aberrations are common, and the customary social order breaks down.[29] Such findings, of course, are not necessarily applicable to humans.

Other researchers have attributed "crowding" not just to the number of people in a given space, but also to the amount of architectural and psychological privacy each person has. Eric Sundstrom, in a study of open offices conducted at the University of Tennessee, concluded that such crowding can produce discomfort and downgrade job performance.[30] Moreover, "crowding" depends upon the type of work being done; Sundstrom also concluded that as work complexity increased, the desired amount of social contact decreased.

THE COFFEE BREAK

For all of the talk about good nutrition, the idea hasn't yet reached the office. If you look at the eating and drinking habits of the vast majority of office workers, it's no wonder that there are complaints about fatigue, stress, headaches, and other ailments.

Consider the office coffee break. Even its name has institutionalized a beverage of questionable repute. Coffee may well be the most popular American beverage, but it is far from the most healthful one. In the last few years, there has been a series of findings about the health effects of caffeine. The evidence indicates that a cup or two of coffee a day may be perfectly all right for most people, but more than that could cause trouble. For example:

• People who drink coffee may be at double or triple the risk of developing pancreatic cancer, a rare but lethal disease, according to epidemiologists at the Harvard School of Public Health. The researchers estimated that "slightly more than 50 percent" of pancreatic cancer cases may be attributed to coffee consumption. The risk was much higher in women than in men, and rose in proportion to the amount of coffee consumed.[31]

• Caffeine has been linked to withdrawal symptoms that appear when a person's customary intake of coffee is cut off. Among the reported effects of caffeine withdrawal are headaches, irritability, drowsiness, and lethargy. A group of researchers at Centre College of Kentucky added anxiety and muscle tension to that list after a study of college students found that "even a brief abstinence may produce anxiety in the regular user."[32]

• Another study found that high doses of caffeine can produce "symptoms that are indistinguishable from those of anxiety neurosis." Nervousness, irritability, rapid heart rate, and muscle twitchings can result from maintaining a high intake of caffeine.[33]

Stimulants such as coffee and tea cause an elevator-like reaction in the body — they take you from level ground up to the penthouse, then down into the basement. Caffeine causes a rise in nearly all vital body functions: it stimulates the brain, widens coronary arteries, increases the heart rate, increases secretion of stomach acids, steps up kidney and bladder action, and increases the overall metabolic rate. It also causes a rapid rise in blood sugar. Then, the process is reversed: everything comes tumbling down, resulting in fatigue, anxiety, and irritability.

If you add another common component of the office coffee break — a donut, sweet roll, or other "junk" food — it enhances the process, causing blood sugar to shoot up even higher and faster. And the higher it goes, the farther it falls. Tobacco smoke is another contributor. A study at Dalhousie University in Halifax, Nova Scotia, found that the more you smoke, the more coffee you want, since cigarette smoke speeds up the elimination of caffeine, which, in turn, steps up the demand for additional stimulants.[34]

Caffeine doesn't come only from coffee, although that is the most potent source. Here is the caffeine content of common beverages:[35]

Brewed coffee: 75 milligrams of caffeine per six-ounce cup.

Instant coffee: 50 to 80 milligrams per six-ounce cup.

Decaffeinated coffee: two to five milligrams per six-ounce cup.

Brewed tea: 15 to 45 milligrams (weak), 40 to 80 milligrams (medium), 70 to 110 milligrams (strong) per six-ounce cup.

Instant tea: 50 to 65 milligrams per six-ounce cup.

Cola: 30 to 50 milligrams per twelve-ounce serving.

How much coffee or other caffeinated beverage should you drink in a day? The answer depends partly on your individual tolerance to caffeine. Generally, however, two cups a day is sufficient to fire up your system in the morning and provide a recharge at midday. You might try substituting all or part of your regular coffee blend with decaffeinated coffee, and request that your office coffee machine be supplemented with alternative beverages, such as bouillon or coffee blends that include grain. In addition, high-protein snacks during the day are a healthy alternative to the sweet nothings available from vending machines and newspaper stands.

OFFICES AND EXERCISE

If you were to believe the books and the health club advertisements, you'd think that only executives get "stressed." That's the message made clear by the growing popularity of "executive fitness" that no doubt has been extremely profitable for a number of publishers and health club proprietors. But exercise is vital to other office workers too, particularly those whose principal source of exercise during the workday consists of walking to the photocopier and the lunchroom.

There's no need to make a case that being sedentary is bad and that exercise can relieve muscular and emotional stress. That's well known. Yet the typical office worker gets little exercise during the workday — and typically is too tired, or has family responsibilities, after work and on weekends to establish a sensible exercise routine. And few offices support extracurricular physical activity during the workday: While on a coffee break, there may be plenty of space to drink coffee or to have a cigarette, but you'll be hard-pressed to find an open area to perform five minutes of stretching exercises that might help you stay more alert at your desk. Exercise in the office just isn't a sanctioned activity. And few offices provide bicycle racks and lockers for those who brave the traffic and air pollution to propel themselves to work each day. It's a frustrating situation for office workers who happen to consider exercise an important part of their daily routines.

That attitude is changing a little, but far from enough. A few large corporations have added exercise facilities to their offices, and many others have sponsored employees' memberships in downtown health clubs. A handful of progressive companies even offer relaxation courses to employees. But companies need not even construct gyms or pay for expensive memberships, although those amenities certainly are welcome. All that's really needed is a small carpeted space for workers to do a few minutes of stretching exercises.

That, too, is beginning to appear in a small number of offices, although most office managers and executives still feel that it's more trouble than it's worth. Shelley Liebman, who gives exercise classes in offices in the Washington, D.C., area, knows well the frustration: "Many offices have conference rooms or other spaces that could easily be used for informal exercises. But most office managers I've talked to haven't the foggiest notion that a few minutes of exercise can make their employees far more efficient. The general attitude is that the whole affair is one big hassle, one they could easily do without."

There are indications that labor unions are beginning

to fill this gap. In New York, for example, about twenty United Store Workers union members with high blood pressure have participated in a technique called "cue-controlled relaxation." A psychologist teaches them to alternately tense and relax their muscles as a method of learning how to relax. Such techniques are badly needed in a country where about a third of the work force suffers from high blood pressure, a disease that results in some 27 million lost work days annually.[35]

Whether or not there's a formal program, there are a number of simple exercises that workers can do at the office to relax or to stay in shape; many can be done while sitting at a desk. Some suggestions for stretching and relaxation exercises are offered in the Appendix of this book.

'MONDAY MORNING SICKNESS'

In recent years, researchers have become fascinated with the relationship between stress and specific time periods. For example, a 1976 study of clerical workers at a Canadian university correlated stress and fatigue with times of day and days of the week. In a 40-day assessment period, it was found that the workers felt best on Fridays, next best on Mondays, and worst on Tuesdays. During the course of a day, fatigue and stress were lowest during the first hour of work, increasing only slightly until lunch. There was a progressively steeper increase after lunch, peaking at day's end.[36]

Scientists also have observed what has come to be known as "Monday Morning Sickness." A project completed in 1980 at another Canadian university studied the lives and deaths of nearly 4,000 men over the course of 32 years. They found that fatal heart attacks in men who hadn't any previous evidence of heart disease were more likely to occur on Mondays than on any other day of the week. The researchers concluded, "Reintroduction to occupational stress, activity, or pollutants after a weekend respite may be factors precipitating the arrhythmias that are the presumed basis for sudden death." They suggested that "psychological stress has been related to sudden cardiac death and return to work may serve as a stressor."[37]

ALL IN THE HEAD?

A few years ago, investigators at NIOSH began to observe some mysterious incidents in factories. For example, at a midwestern electronics assembly plant employing 500 workers, 90 female employees from the first shift reported a variety of nonspecific symptoms such as headaches, dizziness, and lightheadedness in response to a strange odor in the workplace. Although environmental testing found some localized concentrations of a few airborne contaminants, there were no pollutants found to account for the outbreaks of illness. Interviews of the affected workers revealed that they complained about more office environmental discomforts (mostly air temperature variations and poor lighting) and job stress (increase in work load, conflicts with supervisors) than the nonaffected workers did.[38]

A similar occurrence took place at a shoe factory, where between 50 and 75 workers experienced headaches, dizziness, and lightheadedness, also in response to a strange odor. Again, there was no explanation for the odor, and interviews with the affected workers found more dissatisfaction with the work environment, more physical and psychological stress on the job, and more stress from financial pressures at home.[39]

Were all of these workers' "illnesses" the result of stress? Were their illnesses primarily "in their heads"? Those are two intriguing questions being asked by industrial hygienists at government agencies and in the private sector. In both of the above cases, the outbreaks were attributed to what has come to be known as "mass psychogenic illness" — one result of stress in the workplace.

The term refers to illnesses that spread suddenly throughout a group of people, but for which no apparent source can be identified. The outbreak is usually precipitated by some form of psychological stress, and affected individuals attribute their illness to a mysterious agent, such as a bug bite or a strange odor. The vast majority of cases involve women.

The notion of psychologically induced illness is foreign to most people, including most employers and supervisors, who tend to regard health complaints for which there are no obvious and specific causes as something just short of worker rebellion. In fact, some mass psychogenic illness cases have occurred in workplaces in which there already were worker-management problems, detracting from the credibility of the workers' health complaints and adding credibility to management's charges of worker insurgency, or whatever.

Until recently, little was known about mass psychogenic illnesses. Over the past few years, investigators at NIOSH and at state health agencies have interviewed more than a thousand affected workers in factories, as well as an equal number of their colleagues who were not affected. The portrait of the phenomenon is emerging, slowly, as is the magnitude of the problem. NIOSH researchers believe that it is an important occupational health problem and that the number of cases is much higher than is actually reported.

"The research on worker psychology has emphasized productivity, almost to the exclusion of everything else," says Dr. Michael Colligan, a NIOSH psychologist who is one of the leading experts on mass psychogenic illness. "We're only recently getting concerned about worker satisfaction and the impact of the job on overall health."

There have been no confirmed cases of mass psychogenic illness in offices — only in factories — although some NIOSH researchers confide in private that they are convinced that they do occur there. Moreover, they say, an increasing number of cases will be uncovered in coming years, as researchers learn more about the illness and as office workers become increasingly vocal about their environments. Moreover, they say, many modern offices are ripe for mass psychogenic illnesses, since the factors common to industrial workplaces experiencing such illnesses also are found in many offices: suspicion of contaminated air, inadequate lighting, temperature variations, repetitive tasks performed at fixed workstations, boredom, poor worker-management relations, role ambiguity, lack of social rapport, and large populations of women.

There is no conclusive evidence as to why women are the most frequent victims of mass psychogenic illnesses. NIOSH and other observers suspect that the conflict between worker and wife/mother produces frustration and guilt. When combined with a stimulus — a strange odor in the air, for example, or any number of strange sounds or sights — sensitized individuals may be provided with an explanation for their discomforts. As more workers become "ill" and word spreads around a workplace, those who previously had not experienced symptoms may develop them in response to the mounting anxiety and confusion. NIOSH studies have found that the first workers to disclose their illnesses are the most seriously affected; as the illness spreads, the symptoms lose potency, although the number of cases gains momentum.[40]

As with so many other office hazards, much more research is needed on mass psychogenic illnesses.

CHAPTER SEVEN

DANGER: OFFICE ZONE

For years, the only hazards in the office were thought to be matters of "safety": falls, fires, paper cuts, spindle wounds, and the like. We now know that those may be the least of the concerns facing office workers. Still, safety is a problem that is inadequately addressed in many offices.

Admittedly, it's not an extremely sexy subject. In the mad rush of the everyday business world, a few bruised knees or strained backs don't raise too many eyebrows — especially in light of the lost limbs and toxic fumes risked daily by blue-collar workers. As a result, the subject of safety has been largely ignored by managers and executives, who consider it to be of little interest. The Los Angeles chapter of the National Safety Council, which attempted a seven-hour office safety training seminar, dropped the course due to lack of interest. "It's just not a popular subject," said John Maxwell, who coordinated the program. "Most corporate executives and office managers are convinced that they never have any safety problems. Nobody wants to look it squarely in the eye."

Other attempts to deliver information on office safety have been just short of ludicrous; they are often sugar-coated and presented as something of a Keystone Kops caper. Consider the following promotional blurbs describing three of the training films on file at the National Safety Council film library:

- **Who Needs Office Safety?** (Color, 13 minutes). While giving a lecture on the uselessness of an office safety

program, a safety director slips, trips, falls, and bangs himself into numerous accidents in his own office.
- **You Always Hurt the One You Love** (Color, 13 minutes). An amusing silent movie spoof is one of the features of this film that points out the basic do's and don't's of office safety.
- **You and Office Safety** (Color, 10 minutes). This film covers the problems of office safety in a unique and different way, covers [sic] all the most common types of office accidents. This film will not only leave your employees laughing, but fully indoctrinated in all phases of office safety.

And so it goes. But office safety is no laughing matter; each year, an estimated 40,000 office workers sustain disabling injuries, and there are more than 200 safety-related deaths, according to the Occupational Safety and Health Administration.[1] In addition, there are countless cases of bad backs, bruises, and skin rashes that go unreported, are not considered "disabling," or are not attributed to the office environment. All told, a conservative estimate of more than $100 million is lost annually in medical and worker's compensation costs; lost-time costs may double that figure.

Unlike most other office hazards, many of these injuries may be blamed on office workers themselves, either because of laziness or negligence. In the pressures of everyday work life, electrical cords are strewed on floors to be tripped over, file drawers are left open to be bumped into, cigarettes are left smoldering in trash cans, and boxes or furniture are improperly lifted, causing back injuries. There are some patterns to the accidents. One study found that age and length of employment were factors in the chances of having a serious accident at the office. The highest rate of injuries was among workers under the age of twenty, followed by the 20-to-29 age group. The injury rate among employees with less than a year's service was almost double that of employees with one to four years' service, and three to four times that of employees with five or more years of service.[2]

Of course, poor design plays a role too. Desks and file cabinets designed with sharp corners may tear pants or stockings; lack of adequate electrical outlets may require awkward positioning of extension cords; slippery stairs, loose carpeting, and the like may result in falls. In many cases, the problems result from work spaces that were never intended to be offices; growing businesses and mushrooming government agencies frequently avoid moving into expensive new spaces, opting instead to turn basements and storage rooms into offices despite the lack of proper lighting and other services in many such spaces.

Another cause of accidents is poor enforcement of building codes, particularly concerning fire safety. A series of hotel fires in 1980 brought to our attention the inadequacies of many cities' fire-safety efforts, ranging from blocked emergency escape routes to missing sprinkler systems to nonworking fire extinguishers. In the modern office, actual flames aren't as much of a concern as toxic smoke from burning plastics and synthetic materials, which are used in a wide variety of furnishings and machines. Despite the sensationalism of Hollywood moviemakers, there has yet to be a "towering inferno" of an office building, although numerous fire officials have publicly expressed concern that such a fire would probably bear tragic results in most cities, due to the lack of proper precautions.

Indeed, the safety problems seem endless. At the New York City Human Resources Administration headquarters, cockroaches have virtually taken over, crawling all over desks, walls, and files. The problem became so severe that a meeting was held by management and the employees' union, an affiliate of AFSCME. The government agency agreed to send in a roach bomb squad. In another Human Resources Administration building, investigators found corridors stacked with boxes, blocking fire exits, elevators, and passageways.[3]

So, "office safety" isn't merely a few tips from a comic training film — it's truly a serious business. The daily injuries sustained by office workers may seem insignificant, compared with those caused by the fierce machinery and dangerous chemicals of industrial life, but they become yet another source of white-collar stress — the stuff from which headaches and heart attacks are made.

Here, then, are some of the areas of concern:[4]

Trips and Falls. This is the number-one accident in offices, according to OSHA. Among the causes are:

- Thick carpeting. It may look attractive, but people wearing cork clogs or gum-soled shoes can trip easily on it.
- Highly waxed floors; loose carpeting, floor boards, and tiles.
- Tracked-in rain or snow, spilled coffee, and other slippery liquids.
- Dropped pencils, paper clips, rubber bands, and paper.
- Electrical cords and outlet boxes.
- "Rush hour," usually at lunchtime and around 5 PM, when everyone is trying to get things done in a hurry.
- Broken or loose stairs.

Back Problems. Chairs are part of the problem (see Chapter Two). Another is improper lifting, a common injury during moving day at the office. Instead of calling for skilled help and the right equipment, some workers try to move heavy things themselves, often with disastrous results.

Some tips for lifting:

- Stand close to the load, with feet spread apart for balance.
- Bend your knees, keeping your back straight.
- Squat down and get a good grip.
- Lift smoothly, using your leg muscles instead of your back.
- When you turn, shift your feet; don't twist your body.
- Set a load down in the same manner; always bend your knees instead of your back.

Electricity. A large percentage of offices — both old ones and new ones — aren't adequately designed for the large number of machines using electricity. As a result, extension cords are used, often without much thought as to the hazards they may pose. One big problem occurs in "open" or "landscaped" offices that are flexibly designed for easy rearrangement of desks. Often, electrical outlets are located in specific locations, either in the floor itself or in boxes mounted on the floor. When desks are moved, the outlets may no longer be located where they are needed.

The result is extension cords strung across the floor, or floor boxes located in the middle of corridors where they can cause tripping.

Make sure that any loose telephone lines and electrical cords are taped down to avoid becoming a tripping hazard.

Electricity, of course, presents a shock hazard when machines are not grounded. "Grounding" means connecting a machine to the ground by way of a third wire in the electrical cord. In the event that the equipment has a short circuit or becomes an electrical hazard, the electricity will flow through this ground wire, preventing an electrical shock. A shock or electrocution hazard occurs when equipment malfunctions and parts become energized, causing electricity to flow through the equipment — and anyone who comes into contact with it. If you are not sure whether your office equipment is properly grounded, contact the building maintenance personnel or an electrician.

You also may get a shock by pulling a plug out by the cord, instead of by the plug.

Another electrical hazard results from plugging too many appliances or machines into the same outlet, overloading that outlet. Adapters that increase the number of available outlets should not be used without checking with a building supervisor or maintenance personnel.

Chairs and Ladders. Another source of falls comes from the improper use of ladders when trying to reach high places. Chairs generally should not be used for climbing, and cardboard boxes and other objects found in the immediate vicinity usually are poor substitutes. This is basic common sense, but it is often overlooked in the attempt to get something done *now*.

When using a ladder:

- Use a good ladder and one that is long enough. Make sure it has no cracks or loose rungs.
- Stay off of the top rungs.
- If you use a stepladder, be sure it's fully open and the spreaders are locked.
- When setting the ladder up, use the "four-to-one" rule: The rungs on a ladder should be one rung-length away from the wall for every four rungs up to where the ladder touches the wall.

Clothing. If you work around moving machinery, such as printing machines or data processing equipment, avoid wearing jewelry, neckties, or anything that could be caught in or on the machinery. Loose sleeves, long scarves, even long hair could pull you into trouble. Avoid floor-length skirts or dresses, or long pants with extra wide cuffs.

Fire Safety. In one small Washington, D.C., consulting firm, a secretary replenishes the photocopier's duplicating fluid, then routinely drops the empty canisters in the trash can. Her boss, a heavy smoker, routinely empties his ashtray into the same trash can. One day, smoldering cigar ashes fell near the "emptied" canisters, igniting a few remaining drops of fluid and causing a small fire that was nurtured by the various papers and other garbage in the can. The resulting blaze destroyed thousands of dollars of office equipment and threatened the lives of everyone. Fortunately, no one was hurt.

Fire damage in offices results from such carelessness, as well as from a lack of safeguards taken before a fire occurs. Despite the use of computers to minimize paper in the office, paper still runs rampant in almost any workplace (the increased use of photocopiers probably has something to do with it). In addition, there is wall-to-wall carpeting (often made from synthetic materials that emit toxic fumes when burning), plastic furniture and accessories (also toxic when burning), and plastic-coated electrical wires crisscrossing about a building — all of which pose a serious threat, since toxic gases, not heat, kill most fire victims. The increased use of office machines, more people per square foot, and more clutter in general create additional fire hazards.

Moreover, open office designs create a greater fire hazard, since flames and smoke can be more easily contained in a fully walled office; and an office containing doors that close can provide a better refuge from smoke and heat for trapped occupants in the event of a fire. Also, the completely undivided ceiling allows an instantaneous flash of fire to take place, if the ceiling is of combustible material.

One of the more dangerous developments in building construction is the use of floor-to-ceiling glass exterior walls, a common construction material for many modern skyscrapers. A fire above the reach of an outside fire hose can spread upward on the outside of the building until there's nothing left to burn; with older, conventional buildings, there is usually an 8-to-10-foot layer of brick between the windows and the floor above, making it more difficult for a fire to spread.

One of the major hindrances to fire safety is the lax enforcement of building codes. In many cities, local governments relax fire-safety building codes — which require sprinkler systems or fire doors, for example — to lower building costs and, hopefully, encourage more busineses to locate there. Even the stricter codes aren't well enforced. "Almost every building fire with heavy loss of life resulted from violations of the codes," said Howard D. Boyd, former fire marshal of Nashville, in an article in the _Wall Street Journal_. "There's no way any fire department can protect people in a building that's inadequately constructed or maintained."[5]

Building owners point to insurance company statistics showing that the chances of dying in an office building fire are one in several million — about the same as being struck by a bolt of lightning. But fire officials say otherwise. They point to a 1980 fire in a large Park Avenue office building in midtown Manhattan, in which 125 firemen were hurt, but no occupants were, since the fire occurred after working hours. Had it happened earlier, fire officials claim that at least 100 to 125 people would have died.[6]

Most fires start small, often as smoldering that goes unnoticed until it breaks out into flames. There are three primary ways to locate fires, notify people in the vicinity, and minimize the risks of damage:

 • **Smoke alarms,** used increasingly in homes, can be placed strategically around the office, especially in locations where smoke may go unnoticed for a period of time.
 • **Automatic sprinklers,** which activate at a certain temperature. These are required in some cities and states,

although they may be missing, improperly located, or simply not working.

● **Fire extinguishers,** located within easy reach, for putting out small fires before they spread. These also are required in most areas, although enforcement is often lax, particularly since most extinguishers must be recharged at regular intervals.

A fourth key step is to have an established plan of action during a fire, including fire drills, if necessary. All employees must be thoroughly knowledgeable of escape routes and locations of alarms and extinguishers, as well as important telephone numbers to use in the event of a fire — or even the smell of smoke.

FIRST AID

Office workers, just like other employees, need to know what to do in the event of a sudden illness or other emergency — even an everyday accident. Of course, it's management's duty to see that first-aid supplies are available, as well as to tell workers where the supplies are located and how to get additional aid, fast. Some firms provide first-aid courses for workers on a voluntary basis, often through the local Red Cross chapter.

A brief printed manual of first-aid instruction, prepared for distribution throughout the office, may be invaluable during the crucial minutes before emergency help can arrive. Topics that should be included are:

● **Falls.** Any serious fall is somewhat shocking to the victim. A helping hand may be all that's needed, but sometimes additional assistance should be provided. In all cases, the victim should rest and relax for a few minutes following a fall.

A serious fall may cause internal injuries or fractures. In such cases, the victim should not be moved more than might be required to prevent further injury. Protect the fall victim from curious onlookers. Loosen clothing, especially at the neck and waist. Cover the victim lightly while awaiting help.

A person unconscious from a fall or other injury

should not be moved or roused. Never try to give food or drink to a person who is unconscious.

● **Cuts.** There are two objectives in first-aid treatment of cuts, punctures, or abrasion wounds: control bleeding and prevent infection. Every cut should be washed immediately with warm water and mild soap, or hydrogen peroxide, if available. Permit a little bleeding; it helps to clean the wound. If bleeding is heavy, a sterile (or at least clean) dressing should be applied and pressure put on the area; don't use puff cotton, which can separate and stick to the wound. Slightly elevate a seriously cut arm or leg to reduce bleeding. Serious wounds, and cuts involving fragments or rusted objects, should be treated by a doctor.

● **Heat Exhaustion.** After prolonged exposure to high temperature and high humidity, an individual may become tired, weak, and dizzy, possibly with a headache, nausea, muscle cramps, or fainting. Move the victim into the shade or to a cooler area; it is best if the victim lies down. Raise the victim's feet eight to twelve inches. If the victim is not vomiting, give clear juice or sips of cool salt water (1 teaspoon of salt per glass) every fifteen minutes for one hour. Stop fluids if vomiting occurs. Place cool, wet cloths on the victim's forehead and body. If symptoms are severe, become worse, or last longer than an hour, seek medical attention.

● **Shock.** Keep the person lying down and warm but not hot; perspiration may be harmful. A conscious shock victim should be encouraged (but not forced) to drink frequent small amounts of fluid, preferably saline (containing some salt) — not alcohol, and nothing very hot or very cold.

Shock as a result of severe injury can cause death, even when the injury itself might otherwise not prove fatal. Therefore, it must be given priority of treatment. The victim of a serious injury may not even realize the susceptibility to shock; as a preventive action, the victim should probably be treated for shock regardless.

● **Electrical Shock.** The first and foremost action should be to remove the victim from the source of the shock. *Do not* touch the person directly until the electric current is turned off or the victim is no longer in contact with it. Otherwise, you may become a shock victim yourself. (Victims who have been struck by lightning may be touched immediately.)

Treat for shock (see above). If the victim is not breathing, give mouth-to-mouth resuscitation (see below).

● **Mouth-to-Mouth Resuscitation.** If the victim is not breathing, take the following steps:

1. Place the victim face up on a firm, stiff surface such as the floor or ground.
2. Quickly clear the mouth and airway of foreign material.
3. If there is no neck injury, tilt the victim's head backward by placing one hand beneath the victim's neck and lifting upward. Place the heel of the other hand on the victim's forehead and press downward gently as the chin is elevated.
4. With one hand on the victim's forehead, pinch the nostrils using your thumb and index finger. Take a deep breath. Place your mouth tightly over the victim's mouth and give four quick full breaths. Then give approximately twelve breaths per minute — one breath about every five seconds until you see the victim's chest rise.
5. Stop blowing when the victim's chest is expanded. Turn your head toward the victim's chest so that your ear is over the victim's mouth. Listen for air leaving the lungs and watch to see if the chest rises and falls.
6. Repeat breathing procedure.

CHAPTER EIGHT

THE FUTURE OF THE 'OFFICE OF THE FUTURE'

As this book goes to press in mid-1981, a ground swell of interest and activity is taking place around the issue of office worker health and safety. The notion of the "cushy office job" is gradually being eroded as new studies uncover a broad range of problems in offices.

The sources of such information are as widespread as the hazards themselves. In the past twelve months, more than a dozen major studies have been released — most of them referred to in the previous pages — by insurance companies, universities, government agencies, labor unions, office worker groups, and various other researchers around the world. And there are many more to come. For example:

• The Women's Occupational Health Center at Columbia University recently received a major grant from the National Institute of Mental Health to study stress among white-collar workers;

• The Communication Workers of America began a project at the University of Wisconsin to study stress among its members;

• The Newspaper Guild and the Mount Sinai School of Medicine have entered into an agreement to conduct a wide-ranging study of the health effects of video display terminals;

• The National Science Foundation is studying the "biomedical, psychological, and social effects of stress" and the "prevention and treatment of stress-related diseases";

• The Wisconsin state government has made its state offices available for use in "human factors" studies being conducted by the University of Wisconsin;

• The Communication Workers of America began a project in conjunction with American Telephone & Telegraph and the Washington, D.C.-based Project on Technology, Work & Character, to study ways to improve work conditions in Bell Telephone offices; and

• The Buffalo Organization for Social and Technological Innovation (BOSTI) is completing the first stages of a massive survey of 10,000 American office workers in government and the private sector, to study productivity and job satisfaction. The BOSTI project, the most ambitious study of office work to date, involves a meticulously designed 56-page questionnaire compiled with help from architects, designers, human factors engineers, and social and environmental psychologists. Among the statements office workers are being asked to rate: "I want a place to lie down during the work day....I work elsewhere because temperature, humidity, or smoke at my work place bother me....My supervisor expresses concern about my welfare."[1]

Activism among office workers has grown as well. Early this year, for example, an agreement was formed between Working Women and the 650,000-member Service Employees International Union to create District 925 (read: *nine-to-five*), a division of SEIU aimed at organizing the nation's office workers. Indeed, there has been rapidly growing interest in organizing secretaries and clericals by many unions; with the industrial labor sector shrinking and the service and information sectors growing, many large labor unions are setting their sights on office workers as the last — and largest — unorganized work force in the country. In addition to campaigns by those unions traditionally representing clerical and office workers — SEIU; Office and Professional Employees International Union; American Federation of State, County, and Municipal Employees; and Communication Workers of America — there have been organizing campaigns started by the United Auto Workers, the International Association of Machinists, the International Brotherhood of Teamsters, and other traditionally industrial unions.

The organizing issues used by such unions include more than worker health, of course. As with most labor movements, money is the number-one issue; also important are job security, promotional opportunities, pension benefits, and other concerns. But there is a growing realization that such issues are not entirely separate from the health effects of office environments; financial pressures and environmental problems can contribute to the same stress-related ailments.

Slowly, the research and the organizing are producing results. For example:

• The Boston-based group Nine-to-Five has been working with many of the 5,000 workers at the massive John Hancock Insurance Company to solve a number of problems. At John Hancock's several office buildings around Boston, many workers experienced problems related to increased automation, producing what a Nine-to-Five survey concluded to be a high rate of psychological stress. At Nine-to-Five's urging, a health and safety committee was formed to ascertain specific problems and to work with the insurance company to find solutions. Another problem at John Hancock was asbestos. Several employees were discovered to be working in what the company had called an "empty" warehouse that later turned out to be contaminated with asbestos dust from deteriorating insulation. Nine-to-Five pressured the company to clean up the pollutant and to screen exposed workers for potential health problems.
• The Philadelphia Project for Occupational Safety and Health (PhilaPOSH) has been conducting "stress management" seminars for public sector workers in the Philadelphia area. The group is working with members of SEIU and AFSCME to better understand and deal with issues like indoor air quality, work pacing, and increased work load. The group also is encouraging workers who have had severe stress-related illnesses to file worker's compensation claims — a practice that remains controversial and largely untested in many states, since such claims have been traditionally used only for physical injuries.
• Twenty lawyers at the Equal Employment Opportunity Commission in Washington filed suit in May 1981 against the General Services Administration on behalf

of themselves and their fellow workers — all of whom work in Columbia Plaza, the wretched office space described in Chapter One of this book. The suit asked a U.S. District Court judge to order the federal government to get rid of the noxious fumes, molds, and fungi workers have had to live with on the job.

To be sure, these efforts represent small steps forward, but such confrontations and educational programs were unheard of just a couple of years ago. A large part of the inspiration for this activism comes from health-and-safety victories won by blue-collar workers over the years. And with the well-oiled organizing machinery of the large national unions entering the white-collar workplace, such issues in offices could be the central labor battleground of this decade.

Meanwhile, activism in the industrial sector continues as well. A number of current trends in industrial health-and-safety campaigns also may be applicable to office workers. As office workers continue to follow in the footsteps of blue-collar workers, other attempts to reduce office hazards may include:

"Right-to-know" movements. Efforts to inform workers about potential workplace hazards have accelerated in recent years, due largely to the efforts of a series of grass-roots "COSH" groups, such as the Chicago Area Committee on Occupational Safety and Health (CACOSH), formed in 1972. Now, more than a dozen such groups exist in major American cities. These groups have taken innovative steps to inform factory workers — and, in some cases, office workers — about the potential hazards they encounter each day, and to suggest remedies to minimize risks. At the Continental Can Company's plant in Clearing, Illinois, for example, CACOSH showed workers how to file a complaint about poor ventilation. Within a week, three ventilation fans were repaired and the ventilation problem eliminated.[2] Office workers clearly could benefit from such self-help tactics. City and state governments are helping in these efforts by passing worker right-to-know laws; in 1981, Philadelphia became the first city to expand the "right to know" about hazardous environmental substances to the general public as well as to workers.

The right to refuse unsafe work. Workers' rights with regard to unsafe jobs were more clearly defined with a landmark 1980 Supreme Court decision. The unanimous decision resulted from a 1974 case against Whirlpool Corporation in Ohio, in which two workers refused to crawl out on a screen from which a co-worker had fallen to his death only nine days earlier. The Court, in its decision, emphasized that the Occupational Safety and Health Act provides a worker with the right to choose not to perform an assigned task due to reasonable apprehension of serious injury, coupled with a reasonable belief that no less drastic alternative than walking off is available.[3] There are certain procedures that must be followed to guarantee a worker's rights under this law, and the Court did not guarantee the right to be paid when refusing hazardous work. The law states that a worker may only refuse to do specific tasks; he or she may not merely walk off the job altogether. The decision did not limit these rights only to industrial workers; office workers may find this law to be a formidable weapon to combat unsafe working conditions.

Compensation for "chronic" hazards. Traditionally, worker compensation was paid only for "acute" injuries or illnesses — those that were immediately relatable to a specific incident or accident, such as a broken leg from a fall, a lost limb from an accident, or respiratory illnesses that occurred immediately after breathing a recognized irritating substance. Increasingly, workers with chronic (long-term) injuries also are being deemed eligible to receive compensation. Sometimes the injury or illness results from incidents that happened many years before, or that took place gradually and subtly over years or decades. One landmark ruling took place in early 1981, when a New York state workers' compensation board awarded $29,000 to the widow of a radio technician who died as a result of chronic exposure to microwave radiation; the worker, who died in 1974, had worked since 1930 on a microwave transmission tower atop the Empire State Building.[4] The ruling was the first to acknowledge "microwave sickness" as a cause of death, but it also was one of the first rulings that acknowledged a work-related injury that occurred over an extremely long period of time.

MAKING THE WORKPLACE WORK

The office health-and-safety movement is part of a larger national focus on the "quality of working life," or QWL, as it has come to be known. The movement rejects the adversarial approach to management, opting for increased worker involvement in day-to-day decisions, which add to worker satisfaction as well as to productivity. As described in an optimistic special report featured in the May 11, 1981, issue of *Business Week:*[5]

> A more enlightened view of worker psychology has taken hold today. It stresses that most people want to be productive and will — given the proper incentives and a climate of labor-management trust — eagerly involve themselves in their jobs. This calls for a participatory process in which workers gain a voice in decision-making...

General Motors Corporation, considered a leader in accommodating workers' demands for participation in decision-making, is trying a number of innovative approaches. At the GM alternator plant in Albany, Georgia, for example, teams of workers meet weekly to discuss job problems and production schedules. Workers regularly travel with managers to help approve purchases of machinery.[6]

Shaklee Corporation of San Francisco adopted a "self-managed" work team concept when it opened a plant in Norman, Oklahoma, in 1979 to produce nutritional products, vitamins, and other pills. Some 190 of the plant's 230 employees are organized into teams consisting of between three and fifteen members. With a high degree of autonomy, the teams set their own production schedules based on management's volume goals. They decide what hours to work, select new team members from a pool approved by the personnel department, and even initiate discharges if necessary (three workers were fired within the first two years).[7]

This "more enlightened view" also is beginning to take hold within other innovative industrial firms, encouraged partially by the apparent success of the Japanese with such endeavors. And, not surprisingly, this new-found respect for workers' needs has caught on big among the rank and file: they have responded to such forward thinking with increased productivity, reduced absenteeism, decreased employee theft, lower turnover, and other characteristics that make companies run more smoothly and more profitably.

Office managers might look to these blue-collar examples for inspiration. If, indeed, the "office of the future is a recreation of the factory of the past," as many activists are fond of saying, the white-collar workplace will suffer unconscionable levels of ailments once associated exclusively with the factory: increased stress, alcoholism, and drug abuse; decreased productivity and job satisfaction. If lessons are to be learned from the ailments of the factory, there appear to be a number of shortcuts that may be taken in offices to avoid such needless strife.

Actually, much of what many office workers are demanding from their employers closely resembles the "quality of working life" innovations being praised by *Business Week:* work schedules that allow workers flexibility in setting working hours to accommodate individual needs and styles; worker participation in the way a business is run; worker input into job structure; "job sharing," enabling two workers to share one full-time job so that both can spend time with family and still produce income; improved worker-management communications. All of these are increasingly being implemented in factories, although they are still rarely found in offices.

There have been some worthwhile experiments. At the U.S. Department of Commerce, for example, the Project on Technology, Work & Character helped the agency's auditors to assess their styles of work. It turned out that some auditors preferred to work on extremely detailed projects that involved analyzing numbers, while other auditors preferred to work on more subjective evaluation projects aimed at determining whether funded programs are meeting their stated objectives. As a result of this revelation, the auditors decided to restructure their department's work flows in order to accommodate individual preferences and abilities.

In another project, World Bank employees conducted a

detailed analysis of their agency's word-processing needs. Workers' helped to choose a system, design the physical layout of the word-processing workstations, and redesign their work in order to meet the needs of both the equipment and its users most effectively. The workers also suggested that the equipment be leased rather than purchased, so that the computers could be tried out before a full-fledged purchasing commitment was made.

Such innovations, while encouraging, remain few and far between. At the same time, radical changes in the design and functioning of offices continue to be made at an accelerating rate, as computerization is introduced into a growing number of businesses.

Despite the seemingly mad rush to implement "offices of the future," there is no clear evidence that such offices are really an improvement over the "old-fashioned" variety of a couple of years ago. Sometimes, in fact, an apparent improvement in communications can create more problems than it solves. At the offices of the U.S. Army's Development and Readiness Command in Washington, for example, electronic mail has made message writing so easy that people tend to overcommunicate. Lower-level employees get a kick out of sending copies of notes to high-level executives, a feat accomplished by simply pushing a few buttons.[8]

Such problems result from the failure of most businesses to analyze office automation systems independently before — or after — they install them in their organizations. Jim Driscoll, an assistant professor at the Sloan School of Management at Massachusetts Institute of Technology, surveyed several large users of office equipment and found that not one had attempted to measure the effects of the equipment on productivity, relying instead on the analyses provided to them by equipment manufacturers that told them how much good the equipment is *supposed* to do. Driscoll, who has been studying office automation since its earliest days, maintains that "there is little reason to believe the proposed office of the future will either save money or advance organizational objectives." This observation was corroborated by the U.S. General Accounting Office, the investigative arm of Congress, which concluded in 1979 that there was no basis for presuming cost savings in the word-processing systems used by the federal government.[9]

One reason for these failures, says Driscoll, is that office automation "promises to decrease the motivation of office workers. Their motivation springs in large part from the nature of the work itself as well as from [workers'] social contacts. An emphasis on maximizing machine efficiency, specialization, and centralization destroys these two mainsprings of worker motivation." As a result, he says, "The office of the future would maximize on machine efficiency by using the computer to gobble up the structured tasks in any office and leave people in only two roles: *bosses* and *garbage collectors*. The boss decides what tasks must be done...and the rest of the workforce picks up the garbage which is left over at the edges of the programmed tasks....Such leftovers have no internal coherence since their sole determining characteristic is that the machine couldn't do them."[10]

AN OUNCE OF PREVENTION

Such evidence suggests that office automation may not be everything that it is cracked up to be. The slick advertising and competitive pressure to "go automated" may have pushed some businesses and corporate departments into purchasing computer equipment that does not serve their best interests, or is even needed. If this is true, executives are paying a high price for these electronic gadgets, and their employees are paying an equally high price in the effects upon their health.

If these health problems are to be cured, or avoided in the first place, there needs to be a rethinking of the cost-benefit approach to designing offices — not just with regard to automation, but with regard to every component of office space, including lighting, desks, chairs, layout, and the actual flows of work and communication throughout an organization. A first step in that rethinking process might be the realization that offices, like people, are individual entities with individual styles and needs. A computer system that works in one insurance company may be inappropriate for another; a prefabricated "open-office" system that improves worker efficiency in one organization may impede productivity in another; "what's good for General Motors" really isn't necessarily best for the rest of the country.

Now, none of this may be particularly pleasing to most company managers. Among other things, this enlightened approach requires a bit of additional hard work when considering new office designs or procedures. But it may well have been the quest for simple solutions — computers that "guaranteed" productivity improvements, for example, or open office designs that promised cost savings through flexibility — that resulted in the inadequacies and hazards in the first place. "The typical business president will look out at his sales office and see 20 or 30 people doing a variety of tasks and say, 'There's got to be a better way to do this,'" says Fred Amport, a management consultant in Chagrin Falls, Ohio. "Typically, he'll go out and look at a couple of computers and make a decision without studying it any further. They make decisions that come back to haunt them several years down the road."

Another frequent mistake is the failure to consider the interrelationships between the various components of office design. The unique lighting needs of VDT operators is one frequently overlooked relationship; another is increased noise that often results from placing typists together in clusters for "efficiency." Chairs, lighting, air quality, and noise have at least as much to do with productivity improvements as the introduction of any new piece of technology or improvement in organizational work flows.

A third mistake is to design work processes around office machines, instead of the other way around. "Designers of current office automation systems...assume that people are lazy and cannot be trusted," says MIT's Jim Driscoll. "Therefore, their systems seek to reduce skill levels required by the organization and to generate information by which operators can be controlled by higher level managers." In what he calls a more "humanistic" organizational structure, workers are assumed to have the potential for self-motivation and control. The idea, says

Driscoll, "is to increase the flow of information to the system operators in order to allow them to utilize and *increase* their skills and knowledge."[11]

Such issues will be debated with increasing frequency in coming years, as we realize that there's more to office efficiency than installing a handful of machines and rearranging office space and processes according to what a relatively small corps of product designers says will maximize efficiency and profits. The well-being of the workers — the users of these systems — is of primary importance, since it is through their enthusiasm and support that efficiency and productivity will be improved.

In the end, it's all a matter of balance: maximum use of office space versus overcrowding; energy savings versus poor air quality and inadequate lighting; improved worker productivity versus work overload; improved organizational communications versus debilitating overcommunication; and all the rest. As obvious as these relationships may seem, they are often overlooked in the never-ending quest to cut costs and improve profits.

The problems of office hazards aren't about to go away; in fact, indications are that they will be getting worse. The boom in office-building construction, the continued "retrofitting" of old buildings into new office space, the accelerating pace of automation, and the ever-present concerns for conserving energy virtually guarantee that the hazards described in this book will become widespread in coming years. But it may not be too late to stem the tide.

What's needed is a massive infusion of information about the problems, so that we may fully understand the human costs and benefits inherent in various office designs. Those new information flows are not about to come from government (at least not the federal government), which is quickly getting out of the occupational safety and health business. Nor will they continue to come exclusively from a variety of "outsiders" — universities, labor groups, and researchers — who have so far offered the most enlightening perspectives on office problems.

The solutions inevitably will come from within offices — from managers, executives, and workers taking a fresh look at some old problems, and from decision-makers being as innovative in addressing the challenges of an organization as in addressing those of a marketplace. For all of the questions and uncertainties that surround the issues of office hazards, one thing seems clear: Life in offices desperately needs to change. And change it will. The challenge will be to mold the "office of the future" into not merely a place for people to work, but into a place that works for people.

APPENDIXES

OFFICE HEALTH & SAFETY QUESTIONNAIRE

Before you can begin to solve health and safety problems in your office, it's necessary to clearly identify them. For this purpose, the following questionnaire was developed by the occupational safety and health staff of the American Federation of State, County, and Municipal Employees, District Council 37, in New York City. You may want to reproduce it on full-sized paper and distribute it to workers in your office or department; you should feel free to make modifications that may make the questionnaire more applicable to your workplace.

When filling out the questionnaire, consider only your immediate work area. If your job requires that you go to a different floor, department, or building during the course of a day, it may be helpful to fill out a separate questionnaire for each of these locations. Don't feel limited by the format of the questionnaire, or by the amount of space provided; some questions require a simple "yes" or "no" answer, others need in-depth explanations.

Name ——————————————————————————————

Agency/Dept/Division ——————————————————————

OFFICE DESIGN

How many people work in your area (that you can see from your desk)?

Do all workers in your area work in an open area?

What size is your office?
   A room with 3 or fewer people
   A room with 4-10 people
   A room with 11-20 people
   A room with 21-35 people
   A room with 36 or more people

Is your desk or any co-worker's within 3 feet of a:
>   Photocopier?
>   Teletype?
>   Stencil machine?
>   Posting machine?
>   Other machines?

Does your office have:
>   Enough space?
>   Not enough space?
>   Too much space?
>   Enough privacy?
>   Not enough privacy?
>   Too much privacy?
>   Other?

ENVIRONMENT
Is your office kept clean?
Are trash cans emptied regularly?
Are floors cleaned regularly?
Are there roaches, flies, mice, or other pests? (specify)

MACHINES (Not incl. VDTs)
What machine(s) do you use 4 hours or more each day?
   (specify)

Do you get any breaks while using these machines? For
   how long?
Do you ever have any ill effects while working these machines (headaches, nausea, eye irritation, dizziness,
   etc.)?
Are liquids, powders, or lubricants used to operate any
   machine? (specify brand name and the label contents)

Which of the following do you use daily?
>   White out
>   Stencil correction fluid
>   Rubber cement
>   Other (specify)

Do you use a photocopy machine?
    If so, specify brand and model
How many hours a day do you use it?
Do you leave the hood open while you work?
Do you look into the light while operating the machine?
Does your machine ever smoke or catch fire?
Do you add toner to the machine?
Does the photocopier room have ventilation?

Are you given thorough instructions for using machines, tools, and equipment?
Are you permitted to work without interference or distractions?
Are "Out of Order" signs posted to identify defective equipment?
Are scissors, knives, and other sharp tools kept closed or put away when not in use?

VIDEO DISPLAY TERMINALS
List brand and model of your machine

How many hours a day do you use it?
Do you use it continuously or with interruptions?
Is the screen easy to read?
Does the screen have an anti-glare surface?
What color is the screen?
What color are the characters?
What color is the wall behind the screen?

Is the brightness adjustable?
Is the keyboard attached to the machine, or is it separate?
Are there blinds or curtains on nearby windows?
Do the characters on the screen appear to flicker?
Do you have to strain to read them?
Do you wear glasses while using the machine?
    Are they bifocals?
How often do you have your prescription changed?

When operating the VDT, do you ever:
        Get irritated or sore eyes?
        Get dizzy or nauseous?
        Get tense or nervous?

What do you like best about the VDT?

What do you like least about the VDT?

STRESS AND FATIGUE
Do you stand all day doing your job?
   Half day?
   2 hours or less?
Do you sit all day?
Does your chair give you good back support?
Do your feet rest on the floor when sitting?

Do you have:
      Varicose veins?
      Backaches or pains?
      Stiff neck?
      Foot problems?
      Other ailments? (specify)

Do you ever lift heavy objects at work?
Does your job make you tense?
   Describe specific symptoms

AIR QUALITY
Does your office have windows?
   Do they open and close?

Does your office have:
   Central air conditioning?
   Window air conditioners?
   Fans or other blowers?

Are you exposed to drafts?
   Is there sufficient air circulation?
   Is the air ever smoky, stale, or stuffy?
      If so, about how many hours per day?
Do you ever notice peculiar odors?
Do you know what the smell is and where it comes from?

Is your office usually:
        Too hot?
        Too cold?
        Just right?
        Too humid?
        Too stuffy?
Can you or other workers regulate the temperature?

How often do you get colds?
        Rarely or never
        Once or twice a year
        Three or more times a year
Do you frequently have:
        Sore throats?
        Stiff shoulders or neck?

LIGHTS AND NOISE
Do you use a window as a light source?
What type of overhead lighting do you have?
        Fluorescent
        Incandescent (bulb)
        Other
Are fluorescent lights covered?
Do you have a desk lamp?
Can you adequately control your office lighting?
Do you get eyestrain or frequent headaches at work?

Are you able to talk in a normal speaking voice while you
    work?
Can you hear others well?
Is your work area
        Too noisy?
        Too quiet?
        Just right?

Are there quiet places in the office to go to when you need
    to concentrate?
When you get home from work do you notice any:
        Difficulty with your hearing?
        Ringing in your ears?

SAFETY AND SECURITY
What are the most frequent causes of accidents:
    Lifting heavy objects
    Tripping or falling
    Defective equipment
    Cuts
    Burns
    Other (specify)
_____
Have there been any disabling accidents recently?
    If so, describe

_____
Are fire exits marked?
Do you have access to a fire extinguisher?
    Do you know how to use it?
Do you have fire drills?
_____
Do you know where the nearest stairs are located?
    Are stairs well lit?
    Are they unobstructed?
    Do they have handrails?
_____
Have there been any fires or explosions?
Are there "no smoking" areas in your office?
    Are they enforced?
Is there a doctor or nurse on the premises?
Is there a well-stocked first-aid kit on the premises?
_____
Does your office have adequate security against intruders?
    Are entrances locked?
    Are restrooms kept locked?
    Do elevators have alarms?
_____
Have there been any security problems?
    If so, describe
Do you know how to locate police or security officers in an
  emergency?
_____

GENERAL HEALTH
Does your company give physical exams or medical tests?
    If so, describe
Are you given test results?
Does your company have a health plan?
    Do you think it is adequate?

Do you or your co-workers complain about:
        Skin rashes?
        Infections?
        Dizziness?
        Headaches?
        Eye irritation/swelling?
        Nausea?
        Swollen feet/ankles?
        Sore throats?
        Chest pain?
        Ulcers
        High blood pressure?
Have women in your office had miscarriages or other childbirth-related problems?

OFFICE POLICIES
Do you have a morning break?
Do you have an afternoon break?

Do you work overtime?
        About how much each month?
Are you paid for overtime?
Do you get advance notice of overtime?

How would you describe the social climate at your office?
        Friendly
        About normal
        Unfriendly
        Other (specify)

    Are there any major disputes between workers and management?
        If so, describe
Is your immediate supervisor generally supportive of what you do?

Below, or on a separate piece of paper, describe any other information about your job, the office environment, and your health that you think might be important.

FILING A COMPLAINT

One method for getting action taken on office hazards is to file a formal complaint with the U.S. Occupational Safety and Health Administration (OSHA), or a similar agency on the state or local level. The federal agency, part of the Department of Labor, was created by the Occupational Safety and Health Act of 1970; the act also established the National Institute for Occupational Safety and Health (NIOSH), OSHA's research arm, which is part of the Department of Health and Human Services.

The Act states that employers must maintain workplaces "free from recognized hazards," and provides for fines for violations, although fines against employers are somewhat rare. But the law also requires OSHA to respond to requests by workers for an inspection of any workplace suspected of being hazardous to employees; federal employees and other state and local government workers are not covered under this law, but may be covered under other regulations.

Any worker can request an inspection by sending a completed complaint form to the nearest OSHA office. (A list of regional offices can be found in Appendix G.) OSHA will keep your name secret if you request. On the day of the inspection, an OSHA inspector will tour your workplace, accompanied by representatives of workers and of management. After the inspection, a citation listing violations and deadlines for remedying them will be sent to the employer and to the person who requested the inspection. The employer must post a copy of the citation for three days, or until the violations have been corrected, whichever is longer. If no citation is issued, OSHA will send the person requesting the inspection a letter stating that no violations were found.

The OSHA inspection can be a formidable weapon for a worker or group of workers who have failed to get action on workplace hazards. Of course, the inspection is limited only to those "hazards" that are visible or otherwise detectable — falling ceilings, noise, fire hazards, broken pipes, or insufficient ventilation, for example.

The OSHA complaint is one tactic in the fight for a safe workplace. There are many others. For example, you may contact your regional NIOSH office to request a "Health Hazard Evaluation" for specific hazards; hazards found by NIOSH inspectors will not be enforceable under the law, but the information found by NIOSH may help build your case to OSHA or to another agency. The ultimate goal is to win the right to refuse to handle any material, to change any procedure, to require the repair of any machine that is hazardous to your health, and to exercise that right without the loss of pay or privileges.

The following suggestions on filing an OSHA complaint are excerpted from *How to Use OSHA — A Workers Action Guide to the Occupational Safety and Health Act,* published by the Occupational Health and Safety Project of Urban Planning Aid, (120 Boylston Street, Boston, Massachusetts; 617/482-6695). The project provides technical and tactical information about the hazards of work to low-income people in Massachusetts who otherwise have no access to such resources.

THE OSHA COMPLAINT FORM

You can get an OSHA complaint form, called an OSHA-7, by writing or calling the nearest OSHA area office (see sample form on the following page). Most OSHA offices will accept telephone complaints only in cases of imminent danger.

There are advantages to a complaint signed by many workers. It can help educate other workers, build support, and counteract harassment from management. Even if you are the only person to sign the complaint, you should still get support from other workers.

The information you provide in the complaint form will probably be the only description of the workplace an inspector will see prior to the inspection. The inspector will base all research, and the plan for the inspection, on the information you provide. If your employer insists that the inspector have a warrant, for example, the complaint

Occupational Safety and Health Administration
Complaint

U.S. Department of Labor

This form is provided for the assistance of any complainant and is not intended to constitute the exclusive means by which a complaint may be registered with the U.S. Department of Labor.

Form Approved
O.M.B. No. 044R1449

Sec. 8(f) (1) of the Williams-Steiger Occupational Safety and Health Act, 29 U.S.C. 651, provides as follows: Any employees or representative of employees who believe that a violation of a safety or health standard exists that threatens physical harm, or that an imminent danger exists, may request an inspection by giving notice to the Secretary or his authorized representative of such violation or danger. Any such notice shall be reduced to writing, shall set forth with reasonable particularity the grounds for the notice, and shall be signed by the employees or representative of employees, and a copy shall be provided the employer or his agent no later than at the time of inspection, except that, upon request of the person giving such notice, his name and the names of individual employees referred to therein shall not appear in such copy or on any record published, released, or made available pursuant to subsection (g) of this section. If upon receipt of such notification the Secretary determines there are reasonable grounds to believe that such violation or danger exists, he shall make a special inspection in accordance with the provisions of this section as soon as practicable, to determine if such violation or danger exists. If the Secretary determines there are no reasonable grounds to believe that a violation or danger exists he shall notify the employees or representative of the employees in writing of such determination.

NOTE: Section 11 (c) of the Act provides explicit protection for employees exercising their rights, including making safety and health complaints.

	For Official Use Only		
	Area	Date Received	Time
	Region	Received By	Formal ☐ Non Formal ☐

The undersigned *(check one)*

☐ Employee   ☐ Representative of Employees   ☐ Other *(specify)* _____

believes that a violation at the following place of employment of an occupational safety or health standard exists which is a job safety or health hazard.

Employer's Name

Employer's Address *(Street)*   *(City)*

(State)   *(Zip Code)*   Telephone

1. Kind of business

2. Specify the particular building or worksite where the alleged violation is located, including address.

3. Specify the name and phone number of employer's agent(s) in charge.

4. Describe briefly the hazard which exists there including the approximate number of employees exposed to or threatened by such hazard.

_____

_____

_____

_____

_____

_____

_____

_____

_____

_____

_____

_____

_____

_____

_____

_____

_____

_____

_____

_____

_____

5. (a) To your knowledge is this condition being considered by any other Government agency, or has it been considered by any other Government agency?

Yes ☐   No ☐

5. (b) If yes, and you know, which Government agency?

6. Has this condition been brought to the attention of the employer?

Yes ☐   No ☐   Don't know ☐

7. Please indicate your desire:

☐ I *do not* want my name revealed to the employer.   ☐ My name *may be* revealed to the employer.

NOTE: It is unlawful to make any false statement, representation or certification in any document filed pursuant to the Occupational Safety and Health Act of 1970. Violations can be punished by a fine of not more than $10,000, or by imprisonment of not more than six months, or by both. (Section 17(g))

Signature _____   Date _____

Typed or Printed Name_____

Address (Street) _____ (City) _____

(State) _____ (Zip Code)_____ Telephone_____

If you are an authorized representative of
employees affected by this complaint, please
state the name of your organization and your title. _____

form will be presented to a judge to justify the warrant; the warrant may cover only the areas in your complaint.

Your complaint should show:

- A clear picture of the hazards;
- That the hazards are a serious threat to the health and safety of workers;
- That the hazards violate OSHA standards;
- That management has known about the hazards for a long time and has done nothing to correct them;
- That you are familiar with OSHA standards and procedures.

According to OSHA, almost anyone — including family members, lawyers, union representatives, or neighbors — can file a complaint about a workplace hazard.

A few other tips on filing the complaint:

- Be organized in your presentation. You can arrange the hazards by type (chemicals, noise, machines, etc.), by work area, or by any other category that fits. Number the hazards.
- Use surveys, grievances, and accident reports, if available, to help back up your complaint.
- Be specific. Fully describe the hazards, including brands and models of machines; names of chemicals, or products in which they are contained; and specific locations of pollutants or other hazards.
- Indicate whether the problems are worse during specific times — times of day, days of the week, etc.

Under the law, you may ask that your name not be revealed to your employer. However, by making yourself known, you may stimulate other workers' interest in the complaint, and in better working conditions in general. You also may be better protected against harassment from your employer if other workers are aware of your case. If you believe that you have been fired or harassed for exercising your rights under OSHA, contact the nearest OSHA office immediately; such harassment is clearly against the law.

Note: It is against the law to make false statements when complaining to OSHA. Violations can be punished by a fine or imprisonment.

OFFICE FITNESS EXERCISES

The following exercises come from Shelley Liebman, who teaches creative exercise classes to workers in offices around Washington, D.C. They are designed to provide strengthening and stretching for those who spend long hours at their desks. Says Liebman: "The idea of exercise classes is scary to many workers, who somehow get the idea that they have to be in shape *before* they do these exercises. That's simply not true. These exercises are intended for anyone. By doing them as many times per week as possible, many office workers will find themselves more relaxed and refreshed at the end of the day, with fewer aches and pains."

EXERCISES AT YOUR DESK

Neck and Shoulder Circles:

● Sitting up, back straight. Lift your shoulders and try to make them touch your ears. Hold for two counts. Let your shoulders drop back down. Inhale as you lift, exhale as you drop. (Really let them drop; don't control the release.) Repeat eight times.

● Sitting up straight, shoulders relaxed. Let your head fall forward, with your chin pointed toward the center of your chest. Rotate your head to the side, ear pointed toward your shoulder. Rotate head to the other side, passing through the center position. Repeat eight times.

● Rotate your head and neck in a full circle — center front, to side, to back, to side. Repeat eight times.

● After eight rotations: head down, lace your hands behind your head, and gently stretch the back of your neck. This helps to release tension that may have accumulated in your upper back.

Lower Back:

● Sitting up, back straight. Imagine that there is a small hole in the back of your chair with a string running through it; the string is attached to your lower back. Press your back into the chair, as if someone is pulling the string. As the string is "released," return to a straight back. Repeat eight times.

● Sitting up toward the end of the chair — straight back, legs extended forward with toes pointing up. Starting with the top of your head, roll down the spine. Extend your fingers toward your toes, head toward your knees. Take hold of your toes (or calves) and gently stretch. This is a good stretch for your thighs, lower back, and neck.

Legs and Feet:

● Sitting up straight, feet flat on the floor. (Adjust your position on the chair according to the height of the chair.)

Legs: Straightening your knee, lift your right leg, then lower it down. Change to the left leg. Repeat 32 times.

● Lift your right leg and circle your foot at the ankle for eight counts. Alternate legs eight times.

Feet: Feet flat on the floor. Lift and lower your heels 32 times. If you like, you can alternate feet, but be sure to exaggerate the arch by pressing firmly into the ball of your foot.

A TEN-MINUTE BREAK

● Feet together, arms relaxed at your side.

● Easy, full breathing. Inhale: count *one-one thousand, two-one thousand...* Exhale, continuing counting. Continue until breathing becomes regular and continuous.

● Stand with feet together, arms raised above your head. Stretch to the ceiling, alternating arms. Repeat 16 times.

● Standing: Right hand on hip, left hand over head. Bend at the waist, stretching left arm over right side. Repeat eight times. Other side eight times. Remember to stretch all the way through the fingertips, giving the side a good stretch.

● Stand with your legs 2 to 3 feet apart, arms out to the side (parallel to the floor). Stretch right hand to left toe. Return to standing. Stretch left hand to right toe. Repeat 32 times.

• Bring feet together, toes pointed forward. Bend your knees slightly and gently bounce, keeping your back straight. Repeat 16 times.
• Straighten legs. Lift your heels off the floor, stretching the balls of your feet, and lower. Repeat 16 times.

CREATIVE JOGGING

Basic:

This is an easy jog in place. During every two jogs, inhale; during the next two jogs, exhale. Continue until jogs and breaths are coordinated.

Variations:

• Jog right foot, then left foot, then right foot, then kick your left foot forward. Continue, beginning with the left foot (right foot will kick forward).
• When you kick add a clap.
• Continue jogging, but allow your feet and legs to go in front of you, to the side of you, and behind you.
• To the same pulse as your jogging, switch to jumping jacks: Jump with your legs out to the side, arms clapping overhead; jump with feet together, arms returning to your sides. Repeat 32 times.
• Gradually build up your stamina. Begin with two minutes of jogging. Add 30 seconds every day.

Remember to keep your breath going; return to basic jogging if you have trouble coordinating your breaths.

FULL-BODY SHAKE OUT

Stand with feet together, arms relaxed at sides; easy, full breathing.

• **Face:** Stretch and relax your facial muscles (mouth, eyes, nose).
• **Neck:** Side-to-side stretches, circles.
• **Shoulders:** Circles, foward and back.
• **Arms:** Continue circles forward and back, but let your whole arm swing (similar to swimming).
• **Hands:** Shake out, making fists and releasing.

- **Rib Cage and Waist:** Moving side to side — bending, stretching, circling.
- **Hips:** Rotate pelvis — side to side, front to back.
- **Legs:** Shake out loosely; let your feet be loose, relaxed at the ankles.
- **Toes:** Curl and uncurl, making "fists" with your toes.

Most important is to just do what feels good, and what releases tension and gives you a good stretch.

OFFICE RELAXATION TECHNIQUES

For all of the physical and psychological stress that office workers encounter each day, few workers are ever taught how to relax at work. And yet, it's a relatively simple procedure that may be done in just a few minutes at your desk (although it may work better in a more private setting).

As the problems of worker stress become more widely known, a growing number of companies and businesses are utilizing "stress management" techniques for their workers, often bringing in outside experts to conduct classes for all employees.

One such expert is Lorraine Rose, a Washington, D.C., stress-management therapist and consultant to such companies as Time-Life Inc., the Xerox Corporation, as well as to schools and government agencies. Below, she offers a few relaxation exercises that can be done during a few spare minutes during the work day:

TENSE AND RELAX

One method of producing relaxation is by tensing a muscle and then allowing it to relax when released. Our muscles work very much like pendulums; when we move them far in one direction (by tensing them) they swing into the other direction (when we let go).

This technique can be practiced with eyes open or closed in any environment: lying down, sitting up, or even standing (except for the leg tensings). You may prefer to practice this in a more private place if you feel self-conscious during the movements.

The key is to focus on the sensation of releasing your muscles. Notice how pleasant the sensations of relaxation feel in contrast to the discomfort of the tension. Hold each tension for approximately five to ten seconds:

- Close your eyes.
- Make a tight fist with your right hand. Hold it, exaggerate it, hold it longer, release.
- Make a fist with your left hand. Release.
- Bend your right elbow, tense your bicep muscle. Release.
- Do the same with your left arm.
- Raise your eyebrows to your hair line. Release.
- Make a severe frown with your brow. Release.
- Close your eyes so tightly that it feels as though your eyebrows can touch your cheeks. Release.
- Make a wide artificial smile. Hold it for 15 seconds. Release.
- Make a distinct facial pucker with your lips and cheeks. Release.
- Open your mouth wider than you ever have before. Release.
- Smile and clench your teeth simultaneously. Release.
- Tuck your head deep into your shoulders, and try to touch your ears with your shoulders. Release.
- Elongate your neck and stretch it high. Release.
- Hug yourself in front with your shoulders. Release.
- Hug yourself behind you with your shoulder blades. Release.
- Make a full large circle with your head, once in each direction.
- Hold your breath for seven seconds and allow the next several breaths to be slow and rhythmic.
- Tighten your buttocks underneath you. Release.
- Lock your knees and lift your legs until the thighs tense. Release.
- Point your toes, first forward, and then flex backwards towards your knees. Release.
- Make fists out of your feet. Release.
- Take a deep breath and a comfortable stretch.

DEEP BREATHING

Deep breathing is particularly beneficial in relieving the feelings of stress and tension. When we breathe deeply we create a feeling of dissipating tension, followed by a feeling of comfort and relaxation. Deep breathing can be practiced anytime, anywhere, in any situation.

• When you inhale, the lower abdomen should be moving outwards. If you are sitting, feel as if you are filling up your lap with your abdomen. If you are laying down, move your lower abdomen up toward the ceiling. If you are standing, move your abdomen out in front of you as if you are exaggerating a weight problem.

• When you exhale, move your lower abdomen inwards toward your lower back.

• Allow your lower abdomen to do all the moving. Your upper abdomen may go along for the ride; however, keep your chest and shoulders out of the process.

• Allow your breathing to move along at a slower pace than you are used to. You usually take 10 to 14 breaths a minute; now try to slow that down to 4 or 5 per minute. This may feel unnatural at first, but you will get used to it. In order to breathe that much slower, allow the beginning of the inhale to move particularly slowly. Otherwise, your abdomen will have extended fully in 1 or 2 seconds, and there is nothing you can do for the next few seconds except hold it out there in front of you; that is creating tension, not relaxing.

• Perceive the breathing as gliding movement and let it continue effortlessly. Count from 1 to 5 during the inhale and again during the exhale. This will establish a pattern of continuity.

MIND RELAXATION

Using your imagination to your advantage can be an extremely powerful and effective method of relaxation. Your body responds readily to the pictures and sensations that you focus upon. The key is to allow your imagination to work for you.

You can practice this technique anywhere that you would feel comfortable closing your eyes. You can participate for as little as one minute or for as long as you can spare:

• Close your eyes gently. Stretch out into the most comfortable position that you can.

• Focus on your breathing; let it originate in your

lower abdomen. Allow the rhythm to be slow and gentle.

• Begin to feel each breath carry you further and further away from the outside environment, so that you feel safe, comfortable, and undistracted.

• Imagine that when you inhale, you are breathing in the ingredients of relaxation. Visualize what this inhalation looks like. Imagine that when you exhale, you are disposing of all the physical and mental tensions that you have been carrying.

• Imagine that you are laying or sitting upon something that is more comfortable than any other surface. (Perhaps you are floating on a cloud or on a raft, laying on a hammock or on a feather bed).

• Imagine that your muscles are losing their tightness and rigidity and are beginning to feel soft and elastic.

• Imagine that any tight or sore parts of your body are being massaged. Imagine that your face is gently being sculpted into the calmest of expressions. Imagine that your arms and legs are so comfortable that you wouldn't want to move them for any reason.

• Imagine that you are being effortlessly transported to an environment that is deeply relaxing.

• Visualize exactly what this place looks like, including the landscaping, the decorations, the plant life, the amount of light.

• Imagine the sounds of that environment and feel yourself responding to their soothing nature. Feel the climate of that environment. If you associate any pleasant tastes with that environment, imagine that you can taste them.

• Remember what it feels like to be so deeply relaxed. Take the time to feel it in every part of your body.

• Slowly and gently bring yourself back to the room where you actually are. Open your eyes.

• Take one more deep breath, filling yourself up with all of the relaxation and energy that you need for the rest of the day.

OFFICE WORKER GROUPS

Most office worker organizations in this country are affiliates of Working Women, the Cleveland-based national organization, but there are a few independent groups as well:

Working Women National Offices:

145 Tremont Street
Boston, MA 02111
617/451-9111

1224 Huron Road
Cleveland, OH 44115
216/566-9308

1411 Walnut Street
Philadelphia, PA 19102
215/564-4268

2000 Florida Avenue, NW
Washington, DC 20009
202/797-1384

Working Women Local Affiliates

Los Angeles Working Women
813 South Hope
Los Angeles, CA 90017
213/628-8080

Women Organized for Employment
88 First Street, 302
San Francisco, CA 94105
415/777-1781

Atlanta Working Women
141 Healey Building
57 Forsyth Street, NW
Atlanta, GA 30303
404/522-5444

Baltimore Working Women
128 W. Franklin Street
Baltimore, MD 21201
301/837-3830

9 to 5
140 Clarendon Street
Boston, MA 02116
617/536-6003

Minnesota Working Women
618 East 22nd Street
Minneapolis, MN 55404
612/870-7045

Women Office Workers
680 Lexington Avenue
New York, NY 10022
212/688-4160

Cincinnati Women
Working
9th and Walnut
Cincinnati, OH 45202
513/381-2455

Cleveland Women
Working
1224 Huron Road
Cleveland, OH 44115
216/566-8511

Dayton Women Working
127 East Fourth Street
Dayton, OH 45402
513/228-8587

Pittsburgh Working
Women
1302 Investment Building
239 Fourth Avenue
Pittsburgh, PA 15222
412/261-3714

Rhode Island Working
Women
100 Washington Street
Providence, RI 02903
401/331-6077

Seattle Working Women
1118 5th Avenue
Seattle, WA 98101
206/624-2985

Independent Organizations

Office Workers of New
Haven
148 Orange Street
New Haven, CT 06510
203/432-3868

Women Employed
5 South Wabash Avenue,
Suite 415
Chicago, IL 60603
312/782-3902

OCCUPATIONAL SAFETY AND HEALTH ORGANIZATIONS

During the past decade, a network of occupational safety and health groups has quietly emerged out of the labor, health, and consumer movements. The first such group, the Chicago Area Committee for Occupational Safety and Health (CACOSH), was set up in 1972 as a training and educational organization. Since then, the "COSH" network has expanded nationwide. The groups, which are typically funded by private contributions, vary in their structure and activities, but most work closely with union locals to hold conferences, seminars, and training programs, and some conduct political activity to support occupational safety and health legislation.

In addition to COSH groups, a growing number of labor unions, universities, and other research groups have joined in the examination of office environmental health. Many of the groups listed below can provide additional information or may be helpful in filing claims regarding office-related problems.

Bay Area Committee for
Occupational Safety and
Health (BACOSH)
The Alameda Labor Temple
2315 Valdez #108
Oakland, CA 94618
415/763-9076

Los Angeles Committee for
Occupational Safety and
Health (LACOSH)
13013 Morningside Way
Los Angeles, CA 90066

Santa Clara Committee for
Occupational Safety and
Health (SantaCOSH)
655 Castro Street
Mountain View, CA 94041
408/998-4050

Chicago Area Committee for
Occupational Safety and
Health (CACOSH)
542 South Dearborn #502
Chicago, IL 60605
312/939-2104

Maryland Committee for
Occupational Safety and
Health (MaryCOSH)
305 West Monument Street
#210
Baltimore, MD 21201
301/837-0414

Massachusetts Coalition for
Occupational Safety and
Health (MassCOSH)
718 Huntington
Boston, MA 02115
617/277-0097

Massachusetts Coalition for
Occupational Safety and
Health, Western Region
(MassCOSH)
134 Chestnut
Springfield, MA 01103

New Jersey Committee for
Occupational Safety and
Health (NJCOSH)
701 East Elizabeth Avenue
Linden, NJ 07036
201/925-1030

New York Committee for
Occupational Safety and
Health (NYCOSH)
32 Union Square, #404
New York, NY 10003
212/674-1595

Western New York Council
for Occupational Safety and
Health (WNYCOSH)
343 Huntington Avenue
Buffalo, NY 14214
716/856-6622

Rochester Council for
Occupational Safety and
Health (ROCOSH)
18 Wellington Avenue
Rochester, NY 14611

Allegheny Council for
Occupational Safety and
Health (ALCOSH)
Jamestown Labor Council
PO Box 184
Jamestown, NY 14701
716/664-2590

Oneida-Herkimer Council for
Occupational Safety and
Health (OHCOSH)
Central New York Labor
Agency
239 Genessee Street
Utica, NY 13501
315/735-6101

Central New York Council
for Occupational Safety and
Health (CNYCOSH)
119 Sherman Street
Watertown, NY 13601
315/782-3771

North Carolina Occupational
Safety and Health Project
(NCOSH)
PO Box 2514
Durham, NC 27705
919/286-2276

Philadelphia Area Project on
Occupational Safety and
Health (PhilaPOSH)
1321 Arch Street, Room 607
Philadelphia, PA 19107
215/568-5188

Rhode Island Committee on
Occupational Safety and
Health (RICOSH)
371 Broadway
Providence, RI 02909
401/751-2015

Tennessee Committee on
Occupational Safety and
Health (TNCOSH)
% Center for Health Services
Station 17
Vanderbilt Medical Center
Nashville, TN 37232
615/322-4773

Washington Occupational
Health Resource Center
Box 18371
Seattle, WA 98118
206/762-7288

Kanawha Valley Coalition for
Occupational Safety and
Health (KVCOSH)
PO Box 3062
Charleston, WV 25331
304/925-6664

Wisconsin Committee for
Occupational Safety and
Health (WICOSH)
2468 West Juneau
Milwaukee, WI 53233
414/643-0928

Washington Area Committee on
Occupational Safety and Health
(WACOSH)
666 11th Street NW Room 1001
Washington, DC 20001
202/638-3385

Labor Occupational Health
Program
2521 Channing Way
Berkeley, CA 94720
415/642-5507

Urban Planning Aid
120 Boylston Street
Boston, MA 02116
617/482-6695

Service Employees Inter-
national Union
2020 K Street NW
Washington, DC 20006

American Federation of
State, County & Municipal
Employees
1625 L Street NW
Washington, DC 20036

American Federation of
Government Employees
1325 Massachusetts Avenue
Washington, DC 20005

Communications Workers
of America
1925 K Street NW
Washington, DC 20036

United Auto Workers
8000 E. Jefferson
Detroit, MI 48214

GOVERNMENT OCCUPATIONAL SAFETY AND HEALTH OFFICES

FEDERAL GOVERNMENT
Occupational Safety and Health Administration
U.S. Department of Labor
200 Constitution Avenue, NW
Washington, DC 20210
202/523-8148

National Institute for Occupational Safety and Health
Parklawn Building
5600 Fishers Lane
Rockville, MD 20857
301/443-2140

Regional Offices

Region I (Connecticut, Maine, Massachusetts, New Hampshire, Rhode Island, Vermont)
Occupational Safety and Health Administration
16-18 North Street
Boston, MA 02109
617/223-6710

National Institute for Occupational Safety and Health
Government Center (JFK Federal Building)
Boston, MA 02203
617/223-6688

Region II (New Jersey, New York, Puerto Rico, Virgin Islands)
Occupational Safety and Health Administration
1515 Broadway, 1 Astor Plaza, Room 3445
New York, NY 10036
212/944-3426

National Institute for Occupational Safety and Health
26 Federal Plaza, Room 3300
New York, NY 10278
212/264-2485

Region III (Delaware, District of Columbia, Maryland, Pennsylvania, Virginia, West Virginia)
Occupational Safety and Health Administration
Gateway Building, Suite 2100
3535 Market Street
Philadelphia, PA 19104
215/596-1201

National Institute for Occupational Safety and Health
P.O. Box 13716
Philadelphia, PA 19101
215/596-6716

Region IV (Alabama, Florida, Georgia, Kentucky, Mississippi, North Carolina, South Carolina, Tennessee)
Occupational Safety and Health Administration
1375 Peachtree Street, NE, Suite 587
Atlanta, GA 30309
404/881-3573

National Institute for Occupational Safety and Health
101 Marietta Tower, Suite 1007
Atlanta, GA 30303
404/221-2396

Region V (Illinois, Indiana, Michigan, Minnesota, Ohio, Wisconsin)
Occupational Safety and Health Administration
32nd Floor, Room 3263
230 South Dearborn Street
Chicago, IL 60604
312/353-2220

National Institute for Occupational Safety and Health
300 South Wacker Drive, 33rd Floor
Chicago, IL 60606
312/886-3881

Region VI (Arkansas, Louisiana, New Mexico, Oklahoma, Texas)
Occupational Safety and Health Administration
555 Griffin Square Building, Room 602
Dallas, TX 75202
214/767-4731

National Institute for Occupational Safety and Health
1200 Main Tower Building, Room 1700-A
Dallas, TX 75202
214/767-3916

Region VII (Iowa, Kansas, Missouri, Nebraska)
Occupational Safety and Health Administration
911 Walnut Street, Room 3000
Kansas City, MO 64106
816/374-5861

National Institute for Occupational Safety and Health
601 East 12th Street
Kansas City, MO 64106
816/374-5332

Region VIII (Colorado, Montana, Utah, Wyoming, North Dakota, South Dakota)
Occupational Safety and Health Administration
Tremont Center, 1st Floor
333 West Colfax Avenue
Denver, CO 80204
303/837-5285

National Institute for Occupational Safety and Health
Denver, CO 80294
303/837-3979

Region IX (Arizona, California, Hawaii, Nevada, Guam)
Occupational Safety and Health Administration
11349 Federal Building
450 Golden Gate Avenue, P.O. Box 36017
San Francisco, CA 94102
415/556-0584

National Institute for Occupational Safety and Health
50 United Nations Plaza
San Francisco, CA 94102
415/556-3781

Region X (Alaska, Idaho, Oregon, Washington)
Occupational Safety and Health Adminstration
Federal Office Building, Room 6010
909 First Avenue
Seattle, WA 98174
206/442-5930

National Institute for Occupational Safety and Health
1321 Second Avenue, Arcade Building
Seattle, WA 98101
206/442-0530

STATE AGENCIES

Alabama Department of Labor
600 Administrative Building
64 North Union Street
Montgomery, AL 36130
205/832-6270

Occupational Safety and Health
Department of Labor
650 West International Airport Road
Anchorage, AK 99502
907/276-4855

Division of Occupational Safety and Health
Industrial Commission
1624 West Adams
Phoenix, AZ 85005
602/271-5795

Occupational Safety and Health Division
Department of Labor
Capitol Hill Building
Little Rock, AR 72201
501/371-1431

Division of Occupational Safety and Health Administration
455 Golden Gate Avenue, Room 7232
San Francisco, CA 94102
415/557-1946

Northern California Field Operations Unit
2151 Berkeley Way
Berkeley, CA 94704
415/540-2673

Southern California Field Operations Unit
1449 Temple Street, Suite 106
Los Angeles, CA 90026
213/620-4290

Department of Labor and Employment
251 East 12th Avenue, Room 304
Denver, CO 80203
303/861-4095

Colorado State University
Occupational Health and
Safety Section
Institute of Rural
Environmental Health
110 Veterinary Science
Building
Fort Collins, CO 80523
303/491-6151

Occupational Safety and
Health Division
Connecticut Department of
Labor
200 Folly Brook Boulevard
Wethersfield, CT 06109
203/566-4550

Department of Labor
State Office Building, Sixth
Floor
820 N. French Street
Wilmington, DE 19801
302/571-2710

Occupational Safety and
Health Division
Office of Labor Standards
2900 Newton Street, NE
Washington, D.C. 20018
202/832-1230

Department of Labor
Division of Workers'
Compensation
Bureau of Industrial Safety
and Health
216 Ashley Building
Tallahassee, FL 32301
904/488-2514

Occupational Safety and
Health Consultation Program
Technology and Development
Laboratory
Engineering Experiment
Station
Georgia Institute of
Technology
Atlanta, GA 30332
404/894-3806

Occupational Health Unit
Georgia Department of
Human Resources
618 Ponce De Leon Avenue
Atlanta, GA 30308
404/894-3397

Division of Occupational
Safety and Health
Department of Labor and
Industrial Relations
677 Ala Moana Avenue, Suite
910
Honolulu, HI 96813
808/548-7510

Department of Labor and
Industrial Service
317 Main Street
Room 400 Statehouse
Boise, ID 83702
208/964-2327

Indiana Division of Labor
1013 State Office Building
100 North Senate Avenue
Indianapolis, IN 46204
317/232-2655

Occupational Safety and
Health Administration
Bureau of Labor, State House
307 East 7th Street
Des Moines, IA 50319
515/281-5797

Labor Management and
Employee Standards
Industrial Safety Section
601 West 10th Street
Topeka, KS 66612
913/296-4386

Division of Occupational
Safety and Health
Kentucky Department of
Labor
U.S. 127 South
Frankfort, KY 40601
502/564-2300

Louisiana Health and Human
Resources Administration
Office of Health Services
Post Office Box 60630
New Orleans, LA 70160
504/568-5052

Division of Industrial Safety
Department of Manpower
Affairs
State House, 20 Union Street
Augusta, ME 04330
207/289-3331

Division of Labor and
Industry
Occupational Safety and
Health Program
203 East Baltimore Street
Baltimore, MD 21202
301/383-6830

Division of Occupational
Hygiene
Massachusetts Department of
Labor and Industries
39 Boylston Street
Boston, MA 02116
617/727-3982

Bureau of Environmental
and Occupational Health
Division of Occupational
Health
3500 North Logan Street
P.O. Box 30035
Lansing, MI 48909
517/373-1410

Occupational Safety and
Health Division
Department of Labor and
Industry
Space Center Building, 5th
Floor
444 Lafayette Road
St. Paul, MN 55101
612/296-2116

Division of Occupational
Safety and Health
Mississippi State Board of
Health
P.O. Box 1700
Jackson, MS 39205
601/982-6315

Division of Labor Standards
Occupational Safety and
Health Administration
Department of Labor and
Industrial Relations
Box 449 - 722 Jefferson
Jefferson City, MO 65101
314/751-3403

Occupational Health Bureau
State Department of Health
and Environmental Sciences
Cogswell Bulding
Helena, MT 59601
406/449-3671

Division of Safety
Department of Labor
P.O. Box 95024
Lincoln, NE 68509
402/571-0285

Department of Occupational
Safety and Health
Nevada Industrial
Commission
1923 North Carson Street,
Suite 202
Carson City, NV 89701
702/885-5241

Bureau of Occupational
Health
Department of Health and
Welfare
State Laboratory Building
Concord, NH 03301
603/271-2281

Division of Labor Relations
and Workplace Standards
John Fitch Plaza
Trenton, NJ 08625
609/292-2313

Occupational Health and
Safety Section
Health And Environmental
Department
P.O. Box 968
Santa Fe, NM 87503
505/827-5271, Ext. 250

Division of Occupational
Safety and Health
New York State Department
of Labor
2 World Trade Center
New York, NY 10047
212/488-7760

Division of Occupational
Safety and Health
North Carolina Department
of Labor
4 West Edenton Street
Raleigh, NC 27601
919/733-4880

Division of Environmental
Waste Management and
Research
North Dakota Department of
Health
1200 Missouri Avenue
Bismarck, ND 58505
701/224-2348

Division of Occupational
Safety and Health
Department of Industrial
Relations
2323 West Fifth Avenue,
Room 2380
Columbus, OH 43216
614/466-4124

Occupational and
Radiological Health Service
Environmental Health
Services
Oklahoma State Department
of Health
N.E. 10th and Stonewall
Oklahoma City, OK 73105
405/271-5221

Occupational Health Section
Workmens' Compensation
Board
204 Labor and Industries
Building
Salem, OR 97310
503/378-6796

Bureau of Occupational
Health, OER
Ninth Floor, Fulton Building
P.O. Box 2063
Harrisburg, PA 17120
717/787-6525

OCC Safety and Health Office
Puerto Rico Department of
Labor
Prudentia Rivera Martinez
Building
Munoz Rivera Avenue - 505
Hato Rey, PR 00917
809/754-2134

Division of Occupational
Health and Radiation Control
Rhode Island Department of
Health
206 Cannon Building
Providence, RI 02908
401/277-2438

Division of Occupational
Safety and Health
Department of Labor
3600 Forest Drive
Post Office Box 11329
Columbia, SC 29211
803/758-3080

Division of Occupational
Safety and Health
Tennessee Department of
Labor
501 Union Building, Suite
300
Nashville, TN 37219
615/741-2793

Division of Occupational
Health and Radiation Control
Texas Department of Health
1100 West 49th Street
Austin, TX 78756
512/458-7341

Bureau of Radiation and
Occupational Health
Utah Division of Health
P.O. Box 2500
150 West North Temple
Salt Lake City, UT 84110
801/533-6734

Division of Occupational
Health and Radiation
Vermont Department of
Health
10 Baldwin Street
Montpelier, VT 05602
802/828-2886

Division of OSHA Voluntary
Compliance and Training
Department of Labor and
Industry
205 North Fourth Street
Richmond, VA 23219
804/786-5875

Occupational Safety and
Health Division
Virgin Islands Department of
Labor
Frederiksted, St. Croix
U.S. VI 00840
809/772-1315

Division of Safety
814 East Fourth Avenue
Olympia, WA 98504
206/753-6497

Occupational Safety and
Boiler Division
OSH Consultation Program
West Virginia Department of
Labor
State Office Building 6
1900 Washington Street East
Charleston, WV 25305
304/348-7890

Section of Occupational
Health
Wisconsin Division of Health
Post Office Box 309
Madison, WI 53701
608/266-1704

Occupational Health and
Safety Department
200 East Eighth Avenue
Cheyenne, WY 82002
307/777-7786

FOOTNOTES

FOOTNOTES

Introduction: The Way We Work

[1] "The People Principle," by Shirley Sibert Englund, *Business Week*, April 24, 1978, pp. 24-5.
[2] ibid.

Chapter One: There's Something in the Air

[1] "Clearing the Air on Illness at NBC Offices," *Wall Street Journal*, January 14, 1981.
[2] "Indoor Air Pollution a Growing Problem," *Milwaukee Journal*, June 9, 1980, p. 1; and "Indoor Air Pollution: How Tight is Too Tight," *energy!* newsletter (Washington, D.C.: Alliance to Save Energy), October 1980, p. 3.
[3] *Assessment of the Indoor Environment, Columbia Plaza Office Building*, (Baltimore: Center for Occupational and Environmental Health, Johns Hopkins University), submitted to General Services Administration, December 1980, p. 19.
[4] WHO's primary report on the topic is *Health Aspects Related to Indoor Air Quality*, EURO Reports and Studies #21, (Copenhagen: World Health Organization), 1979.
[5] A good summary of this issue is in *Indoor Air Pollution: An Emerging Health Problem*, (Washington, D.C.: U.S. General Accounting Office), CED-80-111, September 24, 1980.
[6] Richard Duffee, director of odor technology at TRC Environmental Consultants Inc., quoted in "Indoor Air Pollution Raises Risks for People in New Office Buildings," by Jonathan Kaufman, *Wall Street Journal*, July 16, 1980.
[7] "Asbestos in the Office Air," *Job Safety and Health*, (Washington, D.C.: OSHA) Vol. 4, No. 3, March 1976, pp. 13-14; and *Indoor Air Pollution: An Emerging Health Problem*, op. cit.
[8] "The Asbestos Problem," *Harvard Medical School Health Letter*, Vol. V, No. 10, August 1980, pp. 1-3.
[9] Jeanne M. Stellman and Susan M. Daum, *Work is Dangerous to Your Health*, (New York: Vintage Books, 1973), pp. 164-65.
[10] "Toxicology of Urea Formaldehyde and Polyurethane Foam Insulation," by J.C. Harris, et al., *Journal of the American Medical Association*, Vol. 245, No. 3, January 16, 1981, pp. 243-246.
[11] Reported in *Job Safety and Health Report*, (Washington, D.C.: Bureau of National Affairs), March 11, 1980, p. 46.

12 "Xerox Continues Fight to End Rumors of a Link Between Copiers and Cancer," *Wall Street Journal*, May 14, 1980.

13 "Ozone Production from Photocopying Machines," by M.D. Selway, et al., *American Industrial Hygiene Association Journal*, Vol. 41, June 1980, pp. 455-459.

14 *Industrial Exposure to Ozone*," NIOSH, 1973.

15 "Ozone Production from Photocopying Machines," op. cit.

16 From various newspaper accounts, including *New York Times*, Feburary 27, March 3, and March 5, 1981; *Albany Times Union*, February 27 and March 6, 1981; *Syracuse Post-Standard*, February 21, 1981.

17 "Indoor Radiation Exposures from Radon and its Daughters," by Anthony Nero (Berkeley: Lawrence Berkeley Laboratory), LBL-10525, February 1980; and "Human Disease from Radon Exposures: The Impact of Energy Conservation in Buildings," by R.J. Budnitz, et al., (Berkeley: Lawrence Berkeley Laboratory), LBL-7809, August 8, 1978.

18 Information obtained through interviews of Dallas County Medical Examiners Office, Oregon Examiner's Office, and representatives of Liquid Paper, conducted by Working Women. Reported in *Warning: Health Hazards for Office Workers*, (Cleveland: Working Women Education Fund, April 1981).

19 "Photocopy Fuss: This Time IBM," *Science News*, Vol. 118, No. 19, November 8, 1980, p. 294.

20 "Occupational Dermatitis," Data Sheet I-510-81, in *National Safety News*, January 1981, pp. 49-56.

21 ibid.

22 "Allergic Contact Dermatitis Caused by Paper," by Kjell Wikstrom, *Acta Dermato-venereologica*, (49), 1969, pp. 547-551.

23 *National Safety News*, op. cit.

24 "Small-Airways Dysfunction in Nonsmokers Chronically Exposed to Tobacco Smoke," by James R. White and Herman F. Froeb, *New England Journal of Medicine*, March 27, 1980.

25 Reported in *ASH Newsletter*, July-August 1980 (Washington D.C.: Action on Smoking and Health).

26 Reported in "Smoke Signals," *Family Health*, November 1980.

27 Reported in *ASH Newsletter*, September-October 1980 (Washington D.C.: Action on Smoking and Health).

28 Reported in *Executive Fitness Newsletter*, Vol. II, No. 22, November 1, 1980 (Emmaus, Pennsylvania: Rodale Press).

29 "Smoking in the Office: A Burning Issue," by Edward G. Thomas, *Management World*, April 1980, pp. 11-12, 40.

30 *Shimp vs. New Jersey Bell*, Superior Court of New Jersey, Docket: C-2904-75. Donna Shimp's trial is told in depth in *How to Protect Your Health at Work*, by Donna Shimp, et al.

(Salem, New Jersey: Environmental Improvement Associates, 1976).

[31] Reported in *ASH Newsletter,* July-August 1980, (Washington, D.C.: Action on Smoking and Health).

[32] "Hospitals Harbor a Built-in Disease Source," by Eliot Marshall, *Science,* Vol. 210, November 14, 1980, pp. 745-749.

[33] "Early Detection of Hypersensitivity Pneumonitis in Office Workers," by Paul M. Arnow, et al., *American Journal of Medicine,* Vol. 64, February 1978, pp. 236-41.

[34] "Humidifier Lung: An Outbreak in Office Workers," by W.W.Taylor, et al., abstracted in *Journal of Allergy and Clinical Immunology,* Vol. 63, No. 3, March 1979, p. 285.

[35] "The Mystery of Assembly-Line Hysteria," by Michael J. Colligan and William Stockton, *Psychology Today,* June 1978, pp. 93-4, 97-9, 114-17. Other articles on "mass psychogenic illness" cited in footnotes 38-40 in Chapter Six.

[36] *Comfort and Productivity in the Office of the '80s,* The Steelcase National Study of Office Environments, No. II, conducted by Louis Harris & Associates, Inc., p. 20.

[37] "Turned-Down Thermostats Turn Off Workers, Who Face Possible Federal Extension of the Rule," by Michael L. King, *Wall Street Journal,* March 11, 1980, p. 48.

[38] "Union Wins Air-Conditioning Case," *Public Employee Press,* (New York: AFSCME District Council 37), March 1980, p.10.

[39] "When Heat is the Hazard," by Stephen Altman, *Job Safety and Health,* (Washington, D.C.: OSHA), Vol. IV, No. 7, July 1976, pp. 5-10.

[40] ibid.

[41] *ASHRAE Standard 55-74R,* (Draft), March 1, 1980.

Chapter Two: Design Neglect

[1] "Interior Technics: Office Seating," *Progressive Architecture,* (Stamford, Connecticut: Reinhold Publishing), May 1980, pp. 126-131.

[2] Much of this history of offices was taken from "Social-Environmental Relationships in Open and Closed Offices," the Ph.D. dissertation of Yvonne Alice Wathen Clearwater, at the University of California at Davis, September, 1, 1979. ©1979, Yvonne Clearwater; used with permission.

[3] Jacqueline Elder, George E. Turner, and Arthur I. Rubin, *Post-Occupancy Evaluation: A Case Study of the Evaluation Process,* (Washington, D.C.: National Bureau of Standards), NBSIR 79-1780, July 1979.

[4] "We are Becoming a Nation of Knowledge Workers," by Robert Propst, in *Ideas,* published by the Herman Miller Company, Vol. III, No. 1, October 1978, pp. 8-9, ©1978, Herman Miller Inc.

[5] "Corporate Architecture: A Study in Banality," by Paul Goldberger, *Saturday Review,* January 21, 1978, pp. 36-38.

[6] *The Steelcase National Study of Office Environments: Do They Work?,* conducted by Louis Harris & Associates, p. 45.

[7] "Social-Environmental Relationships in Open and Closed Offices," op. cit.

[8] "Psychology of the New York Work Space," by T. George Harris, *New York,* October 31, 1978, pp. 51-52, 54.

[9] "True Tales of the New York Workplace," by Orde Coombs, *New York,* October 31, 1978, p. 69.

[10] "Psychology of the New York Work Space," op. cit.

[11] "Office Evaluation Research: Issues and Applications," by Jean D. Wineman, paper presented at the Center for Building Technology, Federal Workshop Series on Building Science and Technology, "The Office as a Work Environment: The Measurement of Performance," National Bureau of Standards, February 3, 1981.

[12] J. Nemeck and E. Grandjean, "Results of an Ergonomic Investigation of Large-Space Offices," *Human Factors,* Vol. 15, No. 2, 1973, pp. 111-124.

[13] "Post-Occupancy Evaluation: A Case Study of the Evaluation Process," op. cit.

[14] G.S. Daniels, "The Average Man?," Wright-Paterson Air Force Base: Wright Air Development Center, #WCRD-TN-53-7, 1952.

[15] "Interior Technics: Office Seating," op. cit.

[16] "Finding a Chair that Fits," by Jeanne M. Stellman, *Working Mother,* October 1978, p. 140.

[17] "Interior Technics: Office Seating," op. cit.

[18] These recommendations were excerpted, with permission, from "Interior Technics: Office Seating," op. cit.

[19] "Participatory Design," by Robert Sommer, *Ideas,* published by the Herman Miller Company, Vol. III, No. 1, October 1978, ©1978, Herman Miller Inc.

[20] Robert Sommer, *Tight Spaces —Hard Architecture and How to Humanize It,* (Englewood Cliffs, N.J.: Prentice-Hall, 1974), p. 113. This is a classic work on the deficiencies of modern architecture, both indoor and outdoor, from the perspective of an environmental psychologist.

Chapter Three: More Than Meets the Eye

[1] *The Steelcase National Study of Office Environments, No. II — Comfort and Productivity in the Office of the 80s,* conducted by Louis Harris & Associates, Inc., p. 13.

[2] "A Case for Reduced Window Areas," by A.C. Hardy, *International Lighting Review,* Vol. 25, 1974, pp. 90-92.

[3] John Ott, *Health and Light,* (New York: Pocket Books, 1976).

[4] Much of this history of Ott comes from *Health and Light,* op. cit.; and from "They Blight Up Your Life," by John Rothchild, *Mother Jones,* June 1978, pp. 49-52, 56-59.

[5] Lila Shoshkes, *Space Planning — Designing the Office Environment,* (New York: Architectural Record, 1976), p. 84.

[6] "Effect of Ultraviolet Radiation on Physical Fitness," by R.M. Allen and T.K. Cureton, *Archives of Physical Medicine and Rehabilitation,* Vol. 26, 1945, pp. 641-44. Cited in "Lighting for the Elderly: A Psychobiological Approach to Lighting," by P.C. Hughes and R.M. Neer, pre-print of article written for *Human Factors,* 1980.

[7] F. Ellinger, *Medical Radiation Biology,* (Springfield, Illinois: Charles C. Thomas, 1957). Cited in "Lighting for the Elderly: A Psychobiological Approach," op. cit.

[8] "Lighting for the Elderly: A Psychobiological Approach," op. cit.

[9] "The Use of Light and Color in Health," by Phillip C. Hughes, in *Health for the Whole Person,* (Boulder, Colorado: Westview Press, 1980), p. 291.

[10] "The Effects of Light on the Human Body," by Richard J. Wurtman, *Scientific American,* Vol. 233, No. 1, July 1975, pp. 68-72. This is an excellent overview of the effects of light on human physiology, written by one of the leading researchers in the field.

[11] "The Use of Light and Color in Health," op. cit., pp. 286-7.

[12] "The Effects of Light on the Human Body," op. cit.

[13] "Some Effects of Light on the Golden Hamster," by R.P. Feller, et al., paper presented at the meeting of the International Association for Dental Research, New York, March 1970. Cited in Ott, *Health and Light,* p. 151.

[14] "The Effects of Light on the Human Body," op. cit.

[15] "The Influence of Artificial and Natural Sunlight Upon Various Psychological and Physical Parameters of the Human Organism," by F. Greiter, et al., abstract presented at the Seventh Annual Meeting of the American Society of Photobiology, 1976.

[16] "Effects of Spectral Difference in Illumination on Fatigue," by

J.B. Maas, et al., *Journal of Applied Psychology,* Vol. 59, 1974, pp. 524-526.

[17] Ott, *Health and Light,* p. 199-200.

[18] "Fluorescent Lights are Found to Boost Cell-Mutation Rate," by Jerry E. Bishop, *Wall Street Journal,* April 28, 1977, p. 29.

[19] "Ultraviolet Wavelength Regions Implicated in Toxic and Mutagenic Effects of Broad Spectrum Radiation from Fluorescent Lamps on L5178Y Mouse Lymphoma Cells," by Elizabeth Jacobsen and Kenneth Krell, *Mutation Research,* Vol. 62, 1979, pp. 533-58.

[20] Shoshkes, *Space Planning,* op. cit., p. 86.

[21] "The Human Aspects of Office and Display Lighting," part of "Facilities Management" series published by Datapro Research Corporation, October 1978. ©1978, Datapro Research Corporation, Delran, New Jersey.

[22] "Lighting for Productivity Gains," by P.C. Hughes, et al., *Lighting Design and Application,* February 1980.

[23] Shoshkes, *Space Planning,* op. cit., pp. 94-5.

[24] Faber Birren, *Color and Human Response,* (New York: Van Nostrand Reinhold Company, 1978).

[25] "The Lights That Made Pupils Ill," *Commercial Engineering Newsletter,* published by Duro-Test Corporation.

[26] "Office Evaluation Research: Issues and Applications," by Jean D. Wineman, presented at the Center for Building Technology, Federal Workshop Series on Building Science and Technology, February 3, 1981.

Chapter Four: Terminal Illnesses

[1] "300 Jam N.Y. Session on VDT Safety," by Barbara Yuncker, *The Guild Reporter,* (Washington, D.C.: The Newspaper Guild), Vol. XLVII, No. 2, January 25, 1980, p. 1.

[2] "CRTs Pose Health Problems for Operators," by Olov Östberg, *International Journal of Occupational Health and Safety,* November-December 1975.

[3] "An Investigation of Health Complaints and Job Stress in Video Display Operators," by Michael J. Smith, et al., (Cincinnati, Ohio: National Institute for Occupational Safety and Health, Division of Biomedical and Behavioral Science, 1980).

[4] Johansson and Aronsson, cited by Gunnarsson and Söderberg in "Eye-Strain Resulting from VDT Work at the Swedish Telecommunications Administration," paper presented to the Swedish National Board of Occupational Safety and Health (in English), April 16, 1980.

⁵ Ben Esterman, *The Eye Book,* (Arlington, Virginia: Great Ocean Publishers, 1977), Chapter 17: How the Eye Works.

⁶ "Human Factors of Workstations with Display Terminals," (Second Edition) published by IBM Corporation, Human Factors Center, San Jose, California. ©1978, 1979, International Business Machines Corporation.

⁷ "The Physical and Psychological Working Environment At a Terminal-Based Computer Storage and Retrieval System," by E. Gunnarsson and O. Östberg, Report 1977:35, published by the Swedish National Board of Occupational Safety and Health, Department of Occupational Medicine.

⁸ "People with a Stiff Back Should Not Perform Keying Tasks," by S. Carlsoo, *Arbetsmiljö,* 7:23-25. Cited in "Occupational Stress Factors in Secretarial-Clerical Workers," an annotated bibliography compiled by Marvin J. Dainoff for NIOSH, January 1979.

⁹ "Fatigue Assessment on Key Punch Operators, Typists, and Others," by Y. Komoike, et al., *Ergonomics,* 14:1971, pp. 101-09; and "Health Control on Key Punchers, Typists, and Others," by Y. Komoike, et al., *The Sumitomo Bulletin of Industrial Health,* 5:1969, pp. 82-109. Both cited in Dainoff bibliography, op. cit.

¹⁰ Gunnarson and Soderberg, "Eye-Strain Resulting from VDT Work at the Swedish Telecommunications Administration," op. cit.

¹¹ *Race Against Time: Automation of the Office,* (Cleveland, Ohio; Working Women, April 1980).

¹² Wilbert O. Galitz, *Human Factors in Office Automation,* (Atlanta: Life Office Management Association, 1980), p. 39. Galitz, who writes that the information comes from a Xerox "branch office study," cites the following as his source: R.P. Wenig and T.D. Pardoe, *Office Automation Systems,* (International Management Services, August 1979).

¹³ "An Investigation of Health Complaints and Job Stress in Video Display Operators," op. cit.

¹⁴ "Microshock in the Information Society," by Robert Howard, *In These Times,* January 21-27, 1981, pp. 11-13, 22.

¹⁵ Adam Osborne, *Running Wild: The Next Industrial Revolution,* (Berkeley, California: Osborne-McGraw Hill, 1979). Cited in "Women and the Micro Revolution," by Gene Murray, *Spokeswomen,* November 1980.

¹⁶ *The Future of the Office Products Industry,* prepared for the National Office Products Association by SRI International, ©1979, National Office Products Association, Alexandria, Virginia.

[17] Testimony of Andrea Hricko, Health Coordinator, Labor Occupational Health Program, University of California, April 12, 1979, before the State of California Industrial Welfare Commission, Wage Board #3.

[18] *Guide to Health Hazards of Visual Display Units — An ASTMS Policy Document*, (London: Association of Scientific, Technical and Managerial Staffs, undated).

[19] "CSEA Taking Action on VDT Health Hazards," *University Voice*, published by California State Employees' Association, January-February 1981.

[20] Cited in "Health and Safety Bulletin," *Industrial Relations Report and Review*, No. 223, May 1980.

[21] "The Human Aspects of Office and Display lighting," Facilities Management report published by Datapro Research Corporation, October 1978. ©1978, Datapro Research Corporation, Delran, New Jersey.

[22] *Guide to Health Hazards of Visual Display Units*, op.cit.

Chapter Five: The Slow Burn

[1] Paul Brodeur, *The Zapping of America — Microwaves, Their Deadly Risk, and the Cover-Up*, (New York: W.W. Norton & Company, 1977), p. 19.

[2] "Human Injury Relatable to Nonionizing Radiation," by Milton M. Zaret. Paper presented at the seminars on "The Biological Effects of Electromagnetic Radiation," sponsored by The Institution of Radio and Electronic Engineers Australia, Sydney and Melbourne, Australia, August 28-September 1, 1978.

[3] *Vision Problems in the U.S. — Data Analysis*, (New York: National Society to Prevent Blindness, 1979).

[4] *The Zapping of America*, op. cit., Chapter 7: "An Unhealthful Post."

[5] ibid.

[6] *The Zapping of America*, op. cit., p. 14.

[7] "RF Radiation: Biological Effects," by Eric J. Lerner, *IEEE Spectrum*, Vol. 17, No. 12, December 1980.

[8] 'Newsday' CRTs Found Leaking Radiation; Metal Shields Installed to Protect Workers," by Ann Dooley, *Computerworld*, April 24, 1980, p. 2.

[9] "Cataracts Following Use of Cathode Ray Tube Displays," by Milton M. Zaret. Paper presented to the International Symposium of Electromagnetic Waves and Biology, France, June 30-July 4, 1980.

[10] "VDTs Pass Medical Tests," by Bill Radus, *FDA Consumer*, April 1981.

[11] Statement by John C. Villforth, director of the Food and Drug Administration, Bureau of Radiological Health, before the Subcommittee on Investigations and Oversight, Committee on Science and Technology, U.S. House of Representatives, May 12, 1981.

[12] 'Benign' Radiation Increasingly Cited as Dangerous," by Malcolm W. Browne, *New York Times,* October 21, 1980, p. C1.

[13] "RF Radiation: Biological Effects," op. cit.

[14] 'Benign' Radiation Increasingly Cited as Dangerous," op. cit.

[15] "RF Radiation: Biological Effects," op. cit.

[16] ibid.

[17] "FCC Regulation of Personal- and Home-Computing Devices — New Rules After a 3-Year Study," by Terry G. Mahn, *Byte,* September 1980.

Chapter Six: Stressed to Kill

[1] Rexford B. Hersey, *Workers' Emotions in Shop and Home: A Study of Individual Workers from the Psychological and Physiological Standpoint,* (Philadelphia: University of Pennsylvania Press, 1932); quoted in Arthur B. Shostak, *Blue-Collar Stress,* (Reading, Massachusetts: Addison-Wesley Publishing Company, 1980), p. 1.

[2] *Warning: Health Hazards for Office Workers,* (Cleveland: Working Women Education Fund, April 1981).

[3] Hans Selye, *The Stress of Life,* (New York: McGraw-Hill Book Co., 1976), pp. 61-64.

[4] ibid.

[5] "Stress Can Get You Down in the Mouth," reported in *California Dental Association Journal,* January 1981, p. 75; the item is attributed to an article that appeared in the *San Diego Evening Tribune,* date unknown.

[6] "Coping With Stress and Addictive Work Behavior," by Waino W. Suojanen and Donald R. Hudson, *Business,* (Atlanta: Georgia State University), January-February 1981, pp. 7-14.

[7] "Women, Work and Coronary Heart Disease: Prospective Findings from the Framingham Heart Study," by Suzanne G. Haynes and Manning Feinleib, *American Journal of Public Health,* Vol. 70, No. 2, pp. 133-41.

[8] "A Review of NIOSH Psychological Stress Research, 1977," by M.J. Smith, et al., in *Occupational Stress,* Proceedings of the Conference on Occupational Stress, Los Angeles, November 3, 1977. NIOSH publication 78-156.

9 "Sex Differences in Adaptation to Work: Physical and Psychological Consequences," by Laraine T. Zappert and Harvey M. Weinstein; revised version of a paper presented at the annual meeting of the American Psychological Association, Montreal, Canada, 1980.

10 "Stress and the Work Environment," panel presentation at OSHA New Directions Conference, Washington, D.C., December 1980; cited in *Warning: Health Hazards for Office Workers,* op. cit., p. 7

11 U.S. Department of Labor, Bureau of Labor Statistics Bulletin 80-188 (March 1980); cited in *Race Against Time: Automation of the Office,* op. cit., p. 13.

12 "Survey of Working Conditions," conducted by the University of Michigan Survey Research Center for the U.S. Department of Labor, 1971; cited in *Warning: Health Hazards for Office Workers,* op. cit., p. 16.

13 "VDT Operator Expected to Process Over 350 Claims a Day," *Working Women,* (Berkeley, California: California State Employees Association), Vol. 1, No. 2, July 1980.

14 *Warning: Health Hazards for Office Workers,* op. cit., p. 12.

15 Occupational Stress Factors in Secretarial-Clerical Workers," an annotated bibliography compiled by Marvin J. Dainoff for NIOSH, January 1979, p. 55.

16 "Noise Raises Blood Pressure Without Impairing Auditory Sensitivity," by E.A. Peterson, et al., *Science,* Vol. 211, March 27, 1981, pp. 1450-1452; also, "Noises of the Day Boost Monkeys' Blood Pressure," by Philip J. Hilts, *Washington Post,* March 21, 1981, p. A6.

17 Jeanne Mager Stellman, *Women's Work, Women's Health,* (New York: Pantheon Books, 1977), pp. 110-15.

18 Susan T. Mackenzie, *Noise and Office Work,* (Ithaca, New York: Cornell University, New York State School of Industrial and Labor Relations), Key Issues No. 19, 1975.

19 ibid, p. 31. Attributed to *The Economic Impact of Noise,* prepared by the National Bureau of Standards for the U.S. Environmental Protection Agency, Office of Noise Abatement and Control, 1971.

20 ibid, p. 28.

21 "True Tales of the New York Workplace," by Orde Coombs, *New York,* October 31, 1977, p. 69.

22 "Some Effects of Commercial Background Music on Data Preparation Operators," by W.H. Gladstones, *Occupational Psychology,* Vol. 43, 1969, pp. 231-22.

23 *Noise and Office Work,* op. cit., p. 32.

24 "Survey of Office Space Shows That More is Less," *Wall Street Journal*, December 2, 1980. The survey, conducted by Chicago real estate company Howard Ecker & Co., showed that the supply of office space available for rent decreased by nearly 2 million square feet during the year ending December 1980.
25 "The Effects of Social Density," by Winford Holland, et al., in *Ideas*, published by the Herman Miller Company, Vol. III, No. 4, 1979.
26 Robert Propst, *The Office — A Facility Based on Change*, (Elmhurst, Illinois: The Business Press, 1968), p. 68.
27 Robert Sommer, *Tight Spaces — Hard Architecture and How to Humanize It*, (Englewood Cliffs, N.J.: Prentice-Hall, 1974), p. 122.
28 *Crowding in Real Environments*, edited by Susan Saegert (Beverly Hills, California: SAGE Publications), pp. 111-13.
29 *Tight Spaces*, op. cit., p. 35.
30 "Privacy at Work: Architectural Correlates of Job Satisfaction and Job Performance," by Eric Sundstrom, et al., *Academy of Management Journal*, Vol. 23, No. 1, 1980, pp. 101-117.
31 "Coffee and Cancer: A Brewing Concern," *Science News*, March 21, 1981, p. 181.
32 "Caffeine Anxiety," New York Times, September 30, 1980, p. C8.
33 *American Journal of Psychiatry*, October 1974, cited in "Stimulants: Right Idea, Wrong Approach," *Executive Fitness Newsletter*, Vol. 11, No. 26, December 27, 1980.
34 "Stimulants: Right Idea, Wrong Approach," op. cit.
35 "Labor Notes," *Wall Street Journal*, April 7, 1981, p. 1.
36 "Patterns and Correlates of Fatigue Among Workers," by T. Nelson and C.J. Laden, *Journal of Occupational Psychology*, Vol. 49, 1976, pp. 65-74.
37 "Chronobiology of Cardiac Sudden Death in Men," by Simon W. Rabkin, et al., *Journal of the American Medical Association*, Vol. 244, No. 12, September 19, 1980, pp. 1357-58.
38 "An Investigation of Apparent Mass Psychogenic Illness in an Electronics Plant," by Michael J. Colligan, et al., *Journal of Behavioral Medicine*, Vol. 2, No. 3, 1979, pp. 297-309; and "Mass Psychogenic Illness in a Shoe Factory," by Lawrence R. Murphy and Michael J. Colligan, *International Archives of Occupational Environmental Health*, Vol 44, 1979, pp. 133-38.
39 ibid; also, "Mass Psychogenic Illness in Organizations: An Overview," by Michael J. Colligan and Lawrence R. Murphy, *Journal of Occupational Psychology*, Vol. 52, 1979, pp. 77-90; and "The Mystery of Assembly-Line Hysteria," *Psychology Today*, July 1978, pp. 93-4, 97-9, 114, 116.
40 "The Mystery of Assembly-Line Hysteria," op. cit.

Chapter Seven: Danger: Office Zone

[1] "Caution: Office Zone," *Job Safety and Health,* February 1976, pp. 5-12.

[2] "Offices Can Be Hazardous," *Job Safety and Health,* (Washington, D.C.: Bureau of National Affairs), September 26, 1980.

[3] "Roaches Threaten Takeover of HRA," by Geri Ruth, *Public Employee Press,* (New York: AFSCME District 37), November 14, 1980, p. 7.

[4] This section on office safety problems was excerpted primarily from "Caution: Office Zone," op. cit; and *Office Safety,* The Training Institute, National Safety Council, Greater Los Angeles Chapter (used with permission).

[5] "Code Violations Cause Most Big Fatal Blazes, Safety Officials Say," by Richard E. Rustin, *Wall Street Journal,* February 2, 1981, p. 1.

[6] "Fire Officials Fear Skyscraper Holocaust Could Kill Thousands," by Richard E. Rustin, *Wall Street Journal,* January 21, 1981, p. 1.

Chapter Eight: The Future of the 'Office of the Future'

[1] "10,000-Office-Worker Study Measures Job Satisfaction and Productivity," *Contract,* January 1980, pp. 139-43.

[2] "Many Groups Accelerate Efforts to Inform Workers of Potential Work-Place Hazards," by Ray Vicker, *Wall Street Journal,* December 23, 1980.

[3] "Supreme Court Gives U.S. Workers the Right to Walk Off Hazardous Jobs," *Job Safety & Health Report,* (Silver Spring, Maryland: Business Publishers, Inc.) March 11, 1980, p. 43.

[4] "Landmark Award for 'Microwave Sickness,'" *Science News,* Vol. 119, March 14, 1981, p. 166.

[5] "The New Industrial Relations," *Business Week,* May 11, 1981, pp. 84-98.

[6] "Carolina Research Park Illustrates Innovations in Nation's Work Sites," by Janet Guyon, *Wall Street Journal,* April 29, 1981, p. 1.

[7] *Business Week,* May 11, 1981, op. cit.

[8] "Many Managers Resist 'Paperless' Technology For Their Own Offices," by Lawrence Rout, *Wall Street Journal,* June 24, 1980, p. 1.

[9] *Federal Productivity Suffers Because Word Processing is Not Well Managed,* (Washington, D.C.: U.S. General Accounting Office), FG MSD-79-17, April 1979.

[10] "Office Automation: The Dynamics of a Technological Boon-doggle," by James W. Driscoll. Paper presented at the International Office Automation Symposium, Stanford University, March 1980.

[11] ibid.

INDEX

INDEX

JOEL MAKOWER is a Washington, D.C.-based freelance journalist who writes about consumer issues, health, environment, and technology. A contributing editor of *Washingtonian* magazine and a columnist for the *Washington Star,* his work also has appeared in other magazines and newspapers, as well as on radio and television. Between 1976 and 1979, he was co-author of annual editions of *Help: The Indispensable Almanac of Consumer Information,* (Everest House). A native of Oakland, California, he is a graduate in journalism of the University of California at Berkeley.